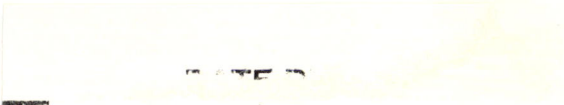

Reforming Health Care:

A Market Prescription

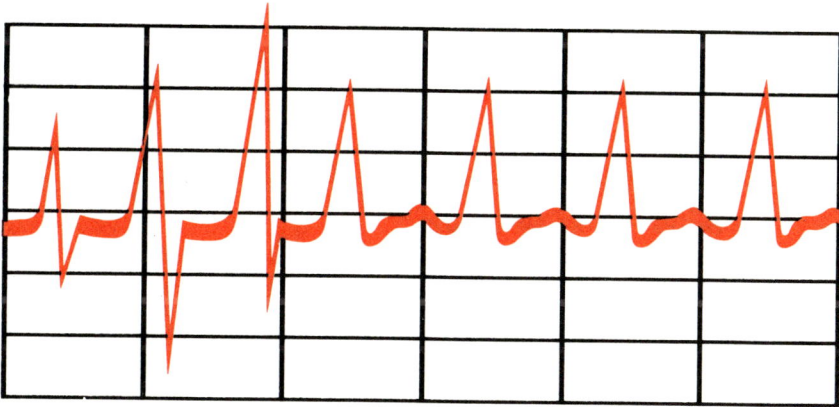

**A Statement by the
Research and
Policy Committee of
the Committee for
Economic Development**

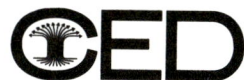

CED

Library of Congress Cataloging-in-Publication Data

Committee for Economic Development. Research and
    Policy Committee
    Reforming health care.

    Includes bibliographies.
    1. Medical care—United States—Cost control.
2. Medical care—United States—Finance.   3. Poor—
Medical care—United States—Finance.   4. Medical
innovations—United States. I. Title. [DNLM:
1. Cost Control.   2. Delivery of Health Care—economics—
United States.   3. Health Planning—economics—United
States.   4. Health Services Accessibility—economics—
United States.   WA 540 AA1 C66r]
RA410.53.C64   1987   362.1'0681   87-11682
ISBN   0-87186-784-2 (lib. bdg.)
ISBN   0-87186-084-8 (pbk.)

First printing in bound-book form: 1987
Paperback: $9.50
Library binding: $11.50
Printed in the United States of America
Design: Stead Young & Rowe Inc.

COMMITTEE FOR ECONOMIC DEVELOPMENT
477 Madison Avenue, New York, NY 10022
(212) 688-2063
1700 K Street, N.W., Washington, D.C. 20006
(202) 296-5860

CONTENTS

Reforming Health Care:

A Market Prescription

RESPONSIBILITY FOR CED STATEMENTS ON NATIONAL POLICY

The Committee for Economic Development is an independent research and educational organization of over two hundred business executives and educators. CED is nonprofit, nonpartisan, and nonpolitical. Its purpose is to propose policies that will help to bring about steady economic growth at high employment and reasonably stable prices, increase productivity and living standards, provide greater and more equal opportunity for every citizen, and improve the quality of life for all. A more complete description of CED appears on page 114.

All CED policy recommendations must have the approval of trustees on the Research and Policy Committee. This committee is directed under the bylaws to "initiate studies into the principles of business policy and of public policy which will foster the full contribution by industry and commerce to the attainment and maintenance" of the objectives stated above. The bylaws emphasize that "all research is to be thoroughly objective in character, and the approach in each instance is to be from the standpoint of the general welfare and not from that of any special political or economic group." The committee is aided by a Research Advisory Board of leading social scientists and by a small permanent professional staff.

The Research and Policy Committee does not attempt to pass judgment on any pending specific legislative proposals; its purpose is to urge careful consideration of the objectives set forth in this statement and of the best means of accomplishing those objectives.

Each statement is preceded by extensive discussions, meetings, and exchange of memoranda. The research is undertaken by a subcommittee, assisted by advisors chosen for their competence in the field under study. The members and advisors of the subcommittee that prepared this statement are listed on page viii.

The full Research and Policy Committee participates in the drafting of recommendations. Likewise, the trustees on the drafting subcommittee vote to approve or disapprove a policy statement, and they share with the Research and Policy Committee the privilege of submitting individual comments for publication, as noted on page 112 of this statement.

Except for the members of the Research and Policy Committee and the responsible subcommittee, the recommendations presented herein are not necessarily endorsed by other trustees or by the advisors, contributors, staff members, or others associated with CED.

RESEARCH AND POLICY COMMITTEE

Purpose of This Statement

U.S. health care is in urgent need of reform. Despite the fact that we spend a higher proportion of our resources on health care than any other country, millions of Americans either lack health insurance altogether or are inadequately protected against catastrophic-level medical expenses. In addition, although there have been innovative successes in the U.S. system, recent public policy changes threaten to retard the innovative potential in our health care system.

Recent proposals for solutions to these problems have fallen short because they have relied on rigid regulations rather than market incentives and because they have looked at these problems as isolated issues instead of interrelated components of our health care system.

The primary motivation for the CED study was our concern about rising health care costs and their effect on the cost of products. We were also concerned about inadequate access to health care services for a significant proportion of Americans.

REFORM BASED ON MARKET INCENTIVES

In this study we offer a comprehensive strategy for reform of U.S. health care focusing on greater reliance on market incentives. Market incentives in public and private health care policies can improve the efficient allocation of health care resources and help us achieve more of our health care goals. We recommend ways to provide for the medically indigent and to make catastrophic or long-term care more affordable. At the same time, we offer steps to control rising health care costs and maintain quality through improved technological innovation.

We believe it is essential that the private sector take the lead in health care reform. Through efficient selection of health care insurance and better management of expenditures on health care, businesses can greatly improve the efficiency of our health care delivery system. Government's major role should be to help provide for the estimated 30 million or more Americans who now lack either private or public insurance coverage.

THE LONG-TERM IMPORTANCE OF HEALTH CARE REFORM

CED's current attention to health care is linked to our continued interest in strengthening U.S. economic competitiveness and ensuring a high standard of living for Americans. A more efficient U.S. health care system would help fulfill both of these goals.

SPECIAL CONTRIBUTIONS

I want to acknowledge the skillful leadership of William S. Woodside, chairman of the executive committee, Primerica Corporation, who chaired the CED subcommittee that prepared this study; and Leon C. Holt, vice chairman and chief administrative officer of Air Products and Chemicals, Inc., who served as vice chairman. I want to acknowledge also the extraordinary contributions of the distinguished group of business and academic leaders who served on the subcommittee and the advisors who gave assistance during the two-year-long process of preparing the study.

To support the work of the subcommittee, CED commissioned a number of research papers on key economic issues by outside experts. These papers, which will be published in a separate volume, are listed on page 113.

In addition, I would like to recognize the important contributions of Project Co-Directors Kenneth McLennan, president and chief executive officer of the Machinery and Allied Products Institute, and Jack Meyer, president of New Directions for Policy. Special thanks also go to Lorraine Brooker, deputy secretary of CED's Research and Policy Committee, and Peggy Morrissette, who, until joining the White House staff, served as deputy secretary of the Research and Policy Committee.

Finally, I would like to thank the corporate and private foundations whose generous support made this publication possible: The Robert Wood Johnson Foundation, The Washington Post Company, American Can Company Foundation, Empire Blue Cross Blue Shield, Pfizer Pharmaceuticals, Rider-Pool Foundation, The Northwestern Mutual Life Insurance Company, SmithKline Beckman Corporation, and G. D. Searle & Co.

William F. May
Chairman
Research and Policy Committee

Chapter 1

Introduction and Summary of Recommendations

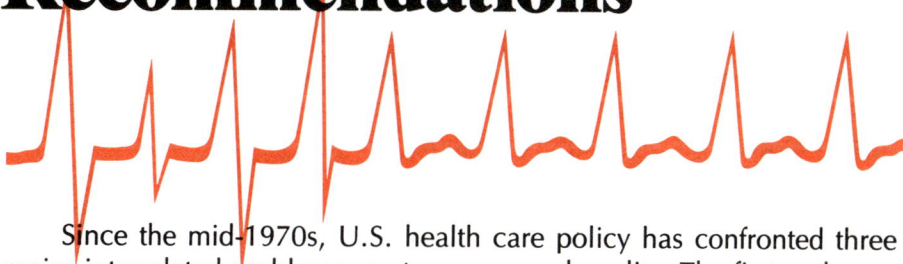

Since the mid-1970s, U.S. health care policy has confronted three major interrelated problems: cost, access, and quality. The first and most visible problem is how to reduce the rapid escalation of health care costs. The primary theme of this policy statement is that such a reduction can be achieved most efficiently through market incentives in the financing and delivery of health care services. The second problem is that the greater reliance on market principles is likely to make it more difficult to assure access to health care for all Americans. Success in solving the problem of escalating costs will eliminate many indirect subsidies, thereby reducing access to affordable health care for a higher proportion of the population. The third problem is that as health care reforms respond to the problems of cost and access, research and development (R & D) and the diffusion of new technologies may be slowed, thus harming the quality of care.

The major purchasers of care, business and government, are becoming much more cost-conscious and are introducing new systems of paying doctors, hospitals, and other providers of services. In response to buyer pressure, these providers are beginning to develop more integrated and cost-effective delivery systems. These changes have helped to control health care costs, but prices are still rising significantly. Indeed, the rate of inflation for medical care was 7.7 percent in 1986, a rate about seven times greater than the rise in the Consumer Price Index. Moreover, the aging of the U.S. population and costs associated with technological innovation may cause health care to claim a larger share of the nation's gross national product (GNP) in the future.

Twenty years ago, health care was a $42-billion-a-year industry, with the government financing 26 percent of expenditures; but by 1985, the industry had grown to $425 billion, with the government financing 41 percent. From 1966, when Medicare and Medicaid were implemented, until 1980, the cost of the combined programs doubled every four years. Although annual increases have slowed considerably in the 1980s, public expenditures on these two programs, financed by payroll taxes and general revenues, continue to grow at a faster rate than overall government spending (of which they represent a significant share).

In the private sector, the cost of employer-based health insurance escalated rapidly during the 1970s. Despite a recent slowdown in the rate of growth in the average annual health insurance premium, employer contributions amounted to $1,549 per person in 1984, or 7.4 percent of payroll.[1] The cost of providing health care insurance for employees and, in many larger corporations, for retirees, along with the cost of payroll taxes for financing government health programs, has significantly increased fixed labor costs. In some industries, this has probably discouraged employment growth.

Many factors determine unit costs of production, and U.S. competitiveness depends on unit costs relative to those of other nations. The rapid increase in health costs appears to be an important factor increasing production costs and decreasing U.S. competitiveness. Indeed, the proportion of U.S. GNP devoted to health care rose from 4.4 percent in 1950 to 10.7 percent in 1985, the highest proportion for any country in the world. Moreover, the United States continues to have a lower productivity growth rate than its major competitors.

The rising share of GNP devoted to health care is not a problem per se. Higher outlays have contributed to a healthier, more productive work force, and the resulting productivity gains have led to a higher rate of economic growth. Thus, focusing only on the *share* of GNP going to health can be misleading.

We should think of health care outlays in much the same way we think of expenditures for education: as an *investment* in human capital. Spent wisely, such outlays stretch the productive potential of the populace and pay dividends in the long run. Moreover, only a small increment to GNP growth arising from additional health expenditures is needed to make such extra outlays cost-effective.

But two conditions must be met for this investment rationale to be justified: First, it is important to direct existing and additional health care expenditures to those services and population groups likely to produce the highest return on the investment. This poses difficult allocation decisions for society. Additional expenditures on prevention of illness and accidents are likely to result in a larger payoff than greater emphasis on acute or long-term care. Should some acute care services be denied if there is a low probability that the patient will recover and be a productive member of the work force? Similarly, GNP will rise more rapidly if most of the increased expenditures are invested in youths and prime-aged workers whose improved health will contribute most to productivity growth. Second, the money must be spent in an efficient way, which requires a system of market signals and incentives that make both the consumers of health services and those who provide them cost-conscious in their use of resources.

Of course, health expenditures are more than economic investments in human capital. They also reflect society's desire to minimize the pain and suffering associated with illness. But in the long run, the ability to achieve the goal of reducing pain and suffering depends heavily on the extent to which investments in health care are economically efficient and produce the return necessary for financing that social goal.

BALANCING BENEFITS AND COSTS

The rapidly escalating cost of financing private and public health care programs is clearly the dominant policy problem facing the U.S. health care system. We believe that by introducing market incentives into private and public health policies, it is possible to deliver services more efficiently. Such a strategy involves a redirection of policy away from the traditional regulatory approach.

Over the years, the growing amount of resources devoted to the health industry has produced substantial benefits. Industries supplying services responded to increased demand by rapidly developing new medical procedures to produce more successful patient outcomes. The higher level of demand encouraged manufacturers of medical devices and pharmaceuticals to develop new products that have provided benefits in excess of the cost to the patients receiving them.

Perhaps the greatest benefit has been that by the 1980s, the vast majority of Americans had access to high quality services. In 1950, only about half of the civilian population was protected by one or more forms of private health insurance; but by 1984, the proportion had risen to 80 percent. The huge Medicare and Medicaid programs guaranteed all the elderly and a substantial proportion of the poor access to basic health care.

The system of providing health care services through a wide range of government and privately financed providers has created considerable diversity in the actual provision of care. This diversity has encouraged different approaches to treating illness in a variety of institutional settings. Compared with more monolithic health care systems, it has given many patients some degree of choice of provider and has probably also contributed to improvements in the quality of services.

4

Despite these benefits, access to health care is still a serious problem for too many Americans, especially uninsured workers in low-wage industries. In addition, many nonworking poor are screened out of public programs by the arbitrary rules of the welfare system. When workers with only minimal insurance protection are added to the uninsured population, between 10 and 15 percent of the population continues to face potential access problems.

Health care markets have special dimensions. For example, people buying health insurance rely heavily on agents — the government, employers, and insurance carriers — for information on the types and availability of health plans. Patients depend on other agents — usually physicians — in making decisions about the need for specific services. Health care consumers are not often sensitive to price, especially when they require treatment for potentially life-threatening or terminal illnesses and accidents. Nevertheless, market principles can operate successfully when health insurance is originally purchased and when individuals require routine medical care. When consumers make these types of decisions, we can expect them to accept a greater share of the financial consequences of their choices.

In the case of most products and services, if individuals are unable to make the purchase, or if they fail to protect themselves against unforeseen risk, they are expected to accept the consequences. But inability to purchase needed medical services can have serious personal consequences that our society is reluctant to impose on individuals. We believe safeguards are needed to assure that those who lack the resources to insure themselves receive assistance. But if an efficient system of safeguards and subsidies is in place, the purchase of health care services can follow the basic principles of a market economy.

As a nation's economy grows, the share of resources devoted to health care will probably increase. Two decades ago, there was an urgent need for the nation to increase expenditures on health care. But the reimbursement system in both the public and the private sectors provided no market signals that would have enabled those paying for the increased expenditures to determine whether the escalating costs were producing any significant improvements in health. As more resources were invested, the additional benefits began to diminish.

By devoting more resources to health services, society used up resources that might have produced a greater return if they had been invested in other activities, such as education, retraining, the environment, new plant and equipment, or national security. For most of the working population, the shift of resources toward the production of health care services included trade-offs in improvements in real wages. Since the shift in resources to the health care sector took place in a sluggish economy with little or no productivity increases, it represented a zero-sum game.

A commitment to two important goals — making health care available to all and ensuring a high rate of medical innovation — will mean that health care expenditures will continue to rise. But the rate of increase will depend on how efficiently the services are delivered. Market incentives can improve the trade-off between cost constraint and greater availability of services and can also reduce, or indeed obviate, the need for the nation to devote a higher proportion of its resources to health care. As economic growth continues, society may, of course, decide to continue to devote more of its total resources to health care, but it must also be prepared to give up the potential benefits of investing these resources in other ways.

MARKET INCENTIVES IN PRIVATE- AND PUBLIC-SECTOR POLICIES

Even with greater reliance on market incentives government will still have a crucial role in improving the performance of health care markets and intervening when market outcomes leave some people with inadequate access to care. Government policies can provide incentives to constrain cost escalation while stimulating innovations and efficiently insuring care for the indigent. Direct subsidies can alleviate the adverse side effects of a more market-oriented approach to cost management. But these effects are not always immediately visible, and the political will to address them could be lacking. Extensive government regulation, however, is not justified.

Greater use of incentives in private-sector health care policies can hold down costs if they make the consumer of health care a more efficient buyer of insurance and if they encourage the use of lower-cost providers. Traditionally, employees have had little choice of benefit plans, and reimbursement followed a cost-plus model that encouraged consumers to select high-cost providers. The introduction of cost sharing makes consumers more aware of the differences among the premium costs of benefit packages, so that they are more likely to consider selecting lower-cost plans. Consumer choice can still be preserved for those who want plans with more extensive services and little or no cost sharing, but the consumer will have to give up some income to pay for the additional premium.

Incentives can also be applied to the use of routine care. By supplying improved information on the cost of services and requiring a variety of checks on whether a service is medically necessary, the employer is in a position to control rising costs through limiting the use of unnecessary services or high-cost providers.

Finally, by adopting market incentives in their health care plans, employers can redirect insurance priorities toward those of greatest benefit to individuals: protection against the high cost of unpredictable accidents or illness. Until recently, many private plans provided first-dollar coverage for routine care but little protection for some forms of catastrophic illness. This meant, for example, that the *entire* cost of a 20-day hospital stay was paid for by the insurance company but no costs were covered after the 20th day. A similar approach was adopted by Medicare when it was implemented in 1966. Insurance for all types of illness should be available, but market incentives will gradually produce a higher priority for protection against catastrophic illness and begin to emphasize coverage for cost-effective preventive services. Greater application of market principles can also constrain cost escalation associated with the traditional reimbursement system, which pays for any services prescribed by the physician.

In recent years, the private sector has begun to adopt market incentives through the redesign of health care plans. We support these changes and favor the strengthening of this trend. Public policies, too, have been reformed to slow down the escalation of government health expenditures. These public and private health care policy changes have reduced the rate of increase in costs, but more extensive use of market incentives will be necessary if health care costs are to continue on a more moderate trend.

IMPROVING HEALTH CARE INNOVATIONS

An important goal of U.S. health care policy is to encourage innovations that will contribute to cost reductions and more effective treatment. There is no reason to believe that the application of market incentives will make this goal more difficult to achieve. Indeed, such powerful incentives are likely to stimulate the quest for cost-saving technologies and encourage the commercialization of successful R & D.

The rapid surge in health care expenditures during the 1970s boosted the rate at which innovations in medical procedures, devices, and pharmaceutical products were adopted. Many of these innovations have proved to be cost-effective. But when the cost of innovation was paid for through a retrospective payment system, it was very difficult to sort out and reduce those technological changes that were *not* cost-effective. Moreover, while we probably got "too much" technology in this sense, we also got too little technology in other areas. For example, there is clear evidence that the rate of approval of new drugs actually declined during the period of rapid expansion in demand.

Some government regulation is, of course, necessary to ensure that new products meet high standards of safety and effectiveness. Market incentives cannot perform these functions on their own. Safety and cost-benefit decisions on new medical products are always made under conditions of uncertainty. Consequently, as the government regulates the use of innovations, it is extremely important that both representatives of the patients who may benefit from the innovations and scientific experts from the government and the wider scientific community participate in the decision on whether to permit the marketing of a particular new medical technology or product.

As in many markets, government support is essential to investment in basic R & D. Much of this government support is funded directly through universities and research institutions. But some basic clinical R & D has traditionally been subsidized indirectly by those who paid above-market prices for routine care in teaching hospitals. Market incentives are now eroding these hidden subsidies. As health care policy moves toward greater use of market incentives, more explicit funding mechanisms will be needed if society is to benefit from sufficient investment in basic medical R & D.

INCREASING ACCESS TO QUALITY HEALTH CARE

The rapid growth of private-sector health insurance has increased access to quality care. But for most of the elderly, for uninsured workers, and for those with insufficient financial resources to pay for needed services, private markets cannot guarantee access. Government policy must fill these substantial gaps in health care insurance. Over the years, Medicaid and Medicare have substantially improved health care access for the poor and for the elderly. Society has, however, a broader obligation: to assist all those who are medically indigent.

The traditional reimbursement system indirectly financed care for some of those who were unable to pay themselves. But this indirect subsidy is beginning to decline because those who are paying the employee health care bill are seeking low-cost providers and are less willing to pay more than the market rate for services in order to cover the cost of uncompensated care. As many of the hidden subsidies for indigent care are eroded, a new method of financing indigent care will be required. CED believes that subsidies should be provided directly to beneficiaries and targeted to actual need.

The challenge for health care policy is to meet the goal of cost constraint and at the same time stimulate health care innovations and improve access to quality care. Greater use of market incentives will eventually provide health care services more equitably and in a cost-sensitive way. Part of these cost savings can be used to finance indigent care. As market incentives are introduced, health care resources will be allocated more efficiently among types of services covered and among groups in society. From society's point of view, if this type of reallocation occurs, the return on the nation's investment in health care will increase. But although health care policies can be designed to increase the overall rate of access to services, a market-driven health care policy will mean that some groups which previously had access to relatively generous health care benefits at little personal cost will eventually have to pay more of the cost themselves or reduce their consumption of services.

SUMMARY OF MAJOR RECOMMENDATIONS

GOVERNMENT INVOLVEMENT AND INCENTIVES IN HEALTH CARE MARKETS

On their own, private markets and changes in employer health care policies cannot provide the entire solution to cost containment, increased innovation, and greater access to care. Although government involvement is necessary, government should avoid regulating the entry of new providers, the services to be provided in benefit plans, and the price of specific services. Market-based incentives are equally important in the implementation of both government and private-sector policies.

MARKET INCENTIVES AND EMPLOYER INNOVATIONS

Since 1970, the average annual cost of providing employer-based health insurance has risen rapidly. In the early 1980s, annual increases of 15 to 20 percent were not unusual for large employers with relatively comprehensive health plans. Part of the cost increase represented the provision of additional services, but much of it was due to the rising cost of existing services.

Many employers concluded that if such cost increases continued, the profitability of the enterprise and its ability to continue to generate employment growth would be affected adversely. As a result, they have revised their health insurance plans substantially, and many are seeking ways to steer employees toward lower-cost providers. Many plans have been redesigned so that the employee now shares costs directly, through coinsurance and deductibles. This is an important step toward encouraging both cost-consciousness and an environment in which providers compete on the basis of price and quality.

CED believes that it is vitally important for employees to be aware of the cost of health care and to share this cost on a fair and reasonable basis. But this cannot be the only, or even necessarily the first, line of defense against escalating costs. Shifting a portion of the total cost of health insurance may not be as important as managing that total amount to achieve the best value for the dollar jointly spent by employees and employers.

Market incentives will be most effective if the consumer has to give up some income at the point when insurance protection is purchased and/or when medical services are actually consumed. Consequently, **CED strongly supports the trend toward greater use of coinsurance and deductibles and recommends that all employer-based plans contain some degree of cost sharing by employees**.

CED also believes that employees will benefit if employers provide some choice of plans with a different mix of benefits. The options can, of course, include no cost sharing when the service is consumed. However, if such a plan carries an additional premium cost, that cost should be paid entirely by the employee. **When multiple plans are offered, it is essential that the employer contribute a fixed dollar amount to the premium, with employees responsible for the extra cost of a more expensive plan**.

Employers can also improve the operation of health care markets by collecting information on providers and giving preference to the most efficient providers. By controlling the utilization rate and the selection of providers, business can use its buying power to stimulate competition on the basis of price and quality.

CED advocates that all businesses, either individually or as part of a business coalition, adopt market incentives and initiate utilization reviews as part of their health care policy. At the same time, businesses should monitor the results of their utilization review process to ensure that employees are not denied access to necessary services simply because the cost appears high.

Traditionally, employer-based plans have emphasized protection for employees and their dependents against risk from routine illness and the potentially catastrophic cost of some acute illnesses. For the most part, however, plans have placed much less emphasis on prevention of and protection against the potentially high cost of treating chronic, long-term illnesses.

CED believes that an effective safety program for prevention of accidents and exposure to workplace hazards has an extremely high payoff in terms of lower health care costs. In addition, although experience with employee wellness programs is incomplete, preliminary results suggest that the benefits of many of these programs exceed the costs. CED also believes that employers and their insurance carriers should experiment with differential insurance rates as a way of encouraging employees to adopt healthy lifestyles.

Neither government nor the private sector has been particularly successful in protecting the small proportion of the population that requires long-term care for chronic illness or acute care involving such elaborate and expensive procedures as organ transplants. In the future, the major burden of financing long-term care for the frail elderly is likely to continue to fall mainly on individuals and their families. Government now provides a safety net for certain types of long-term care expenditures through the Medicaid program. But given the already high level of government expenditures on care for the elderly, it is simply unrealistic to expect that the government can fully fund this type of protection for all who need it.

It is vitally important, therefore, to reform the current system of financing and delivering long-term care through incentives for care at home instead of in institutions along with payment systems that conserve resources. Effective case management and efficient channeling of resources are prerequisites for a long-term solution.

The private sector can make an important contribution to solving the long-term care problem. **CED supports current experiments with social HMOs, continuing-care retirement communities, and reverse mortgages to help finance long-term care for the frail elderly. We also encourage efforts by the insurance industry to market long-term care coverage**.

Employers have a responsibility to educate employees on the value of insurance that protects them against the extremely high cost of long-term care. There is a low probability that such care will be required for the young and middle-aged; but for the *old elderly* (those over eighty), about 30 percent will eventually need some long-term care. With increasing longevity and the aging of the population, there will be an explosion in the demand for this type of care in the next century. **CED recommends that employers begin now to redesign employee benefit packages to include a long-term care option and to offer to contribute to the financing of this option by phasing down the employer contribution to life insurance once an employee reaches age forty to fifty and substituting long-term care insurance. CED further recommends that consideration be given to redesigning Medicare to provide a greater measure of protection for long-term care.**

How to finance access to high-cost innovations such as organ transplants is an issue of increasing importance. It makes little sense to include generous benefits for routine care but deny them for some types of innovations in medical procedures. To finance the high cost of such innovations, **CED recommends that employers consider redesigning health plans to include basic coverage of major medical expenses with an additional rider for coverage of high-cost medical procedures such as transplants**. The additional premium could include a significant degree of cost sharing, perhaps with the amount paid by the employee based on salary.

Greater use of market incentives in health care policy will inevitably highlight the problem of financing indigent care. About half those without health insurance are over thirty years of age and married. Indeed, over half the indigent care population are workers and their families who are ineligible for Medicaid. Many work for small employers who provide no health insurance. We believe that the private sector can play an important role in making insurance available to these workers at group rates.

CED urges employer groups, such as local chambers of commerce and business health care coalitions, working with insurance companies, to assist small employers and individual workers in forming health insurance groups and to extend insurance to those who are currently uninsured. Employers can recognize uncompensated care as a legitimate item in the overhead of providers and assist hospitals in their community that serve a large number of indigent patients. Such actions, we believe, can help to reduce the size of the uninsured population and the cost of indigent care.

INNOVATION IN MEDICAL DEVICES, MEDICAL PROCEDURES, AND PHARMACEUTICALS

Since 1965, the huge increase in demand for health care services stimulated advances in medical technology and procedures. These advances produced significant benefits, but the traditional cost-plus reimbursement system also led to unnecessary use of many innovations. Market incentives and more cost-conscious purchasing by employers will reduce this inefficiency and should limit the proliferation of medical technology without regard to its effectiveness. While avoiding the overuse of technology is clearly necessary, it is equally important to maintain a high rate of innovation in basic medical research and to accelerate the marketing of safe and effective technologies and pharmaceuticals. The underuse of medical research and technology concerns us just as much as its potential overuse.

In the past, advances in medical procedures that emerged from clinical research in hospitals were indirectly subsidized by fee-paying patients and by Medicare. Market incentives in the private sector and Medicare reforms would erode this source of support for basic research. **CED recommends that additional funding be made available through a system of government grants administered through the National Institutes of Health.** Awards should be based on the importance of the research proposal and the quality of the researchers, irrespective of the type of institution at which the research is conducted.

Through the Food and Drug Administration (FDA), the government has responsibility to approve new medical devices before they are marketed.

However, the Health Care Financing Administration (HCFA) must also determine whether new devices will be approved for reimbursement under Medicare. In the past, HCFA has delayed initiating its review for approval until after the FDA has determined that the new device is safe and effective. **CED recommends that the HCFA review of whether the new device will be reimbursed under Medicare be initiated prior to completion of the FDA approval process to avoid unnecessary delays in making new devices available to Medicare patients**.

It now takes one or two years longer for the FDA to approve a new drug than for that drug to receive approval in other developed countries. This has contributed to the declining rate of introduction of new chemical entities in the United States and has encouraged U.S. firms to conduct R & D in their foreign subsidiaries. The government has a responsibility to make every effort to approve only drugs that are safe and effective. However, there will always be some probability of adverse effects under specific conditions, and preventing the marketing of new drugs can also impose costs on those who are denied the drugs' benefits.

CED believes that it is essential to speed up the costly drug approval process. **We recommend that the FDA be required to make greater use of experts from the scientific community outside of government, along with advisors representing patients who may benefit from the new drug**. The final approval decision should remain FDA's responsibility; but if its decision is opposed by a majority of the scientific advisors, the FDA should indicate why it takes a different position. Our recommendation is essentially an adaptation of the regulatory review approach recently authorized for so-called orphan drugs, which are potentially beneficial to only small numbers of individuals suffering from unusual illnesses.

ADOPTING MARKET INCENTIVES IN PUBLIC-SECTOR POLICIES

Most basic medical care is available to those who are unable to pay for it. The Medicaid program provides health insurance to a portion of the poor, and a complex system of hidden subsidies finances care for many low-income individuals not eligible for Medicaid. Of course, some people do not receive care that they need, particularly preventive care, because they lack the means to pay for it. But in a variety of ways, through taxes or hospital and doctor fees inflated above market value, business and its employees have financed a substantial amount of care for the indigent. In recent years, however, these hidden subsidies have been eroded by competitive pressures.

A new strategy for indigent care financing is central to greater reliance on market incentives in private and public health care policies. **It is time to seize this opportunity to target assistance on the basis of need and to subsi-**

dize patients rather than providers. Those eligible for assistance should be given the opportunity to exercise some degree of choice in health care decisions. For these reasons, **CED favors providing low-income individuals with a voucher to purchase basic health insurance**. The amount of the voucher could be based on a sliding scale depending on income.

Such a comprehensive revision of health care policy will require a reform of Medicare because part of the financing of indigent care will be borne by the nonpoor elderly. And systemwide reform will eventually require the substitution of a more complete incentives-based approach to Medicare financing than the current diagnostic-related group (DRG) program.

All groups in society are currently financing indigent care. The CED approach is simply a more explicit and, we believe, more equitable way of ensuring basic medical care for all. A number of options should be considered as ways to raise the revenue for this market-oriented approach. One option is to include a larger portion of Social Security benefits in taxable income. Another option is to raise the tax on cigarettes and alcohol. Workers with relatively generous benefits might also be asked to contribute to the financing of indigent care by including a small portion of the value of their employer-paid health insurance premium in taxable income. **All groups would contribute to the cost of providing care for the indigent. By broadening the base of financing, the cost of covering individuals who now lack insurance would, on average, be very low**.

We recognize that it may take time to implement such a significant change. For the interim, we suggest a series of steps that are not in conflict with the ultimate goal of reforming the current haphazard financing of indigent care. These include (1) a floor on eligibility for health care benefits established by the federal government and (2) reforms at the state level involving both risk pools to cover the indigent and management reforms to encourage the cost-conscious use of health care resources.

Chapter 2

Cost, Quality, and Access: Components of the Health Care Problem

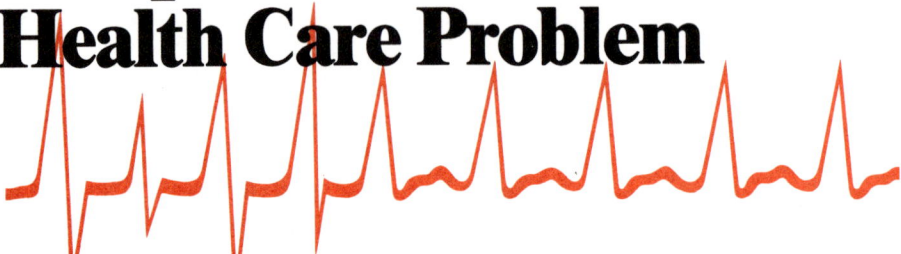

The goals of health care policy involve the complex task of finding ways to moderate the growth of cost while improving the quality of care and increasing access to services. Too often, these goals are oversimplified into an effort to contain costs — at all cost. As important as cost moderation is, it would be a mistake to sacrifice quality or access at the altar of cost containment. It is equally important, however, that the concepts of quality and access not be used as an excuse for ignoring costs or presuming that the purchasers and consumers of care should not question its cost. The key challenge in health policy is to devise powerful incentives to encourage all the actors in the health care system — patients, providers of care, insurers, and those who pay their premiums — to use the system in a cost-conscious manner while maintaining the proper safeguards to assure quality and access.

THE SIGNIFICANCE AND SOURCES OF ESCALATING COSTS

The major pressure to reform U.S. health care policies has been generated largely by the rapid increase in both government expenditures for services and the cost of employer-based reimbursement programs.

As we discussed in Chapter 1, in 1985 about 41 percent of the $425-billion health care sector was financed with government funds (about 71 percent of this was federal dollars), compared with 26 percent of a $42-billion industry in 1965. Americans were spending $1,459 per capita on health care in 1983, compared with $207 per capita in 1965 ($653 in 1983 dollars). By 1985, per capita spending on health care had increased to $1,721.[1]

From 1966 to 1980, the cost of Medicare and Medicaid doubled every four years. In the 1980s, the annual increases have slowed considerably, but these two programs are still major growth areas in the federal budget. Medicare outlays are expected to total $70 billion in fiscal 1987, compared with $7.1 billion in 1970 and $35.0 billion in 1980. The federal contribution to Medicaid in fiscal 1987 is estimated at $26 billion, compared to $2.7 billion in 1970 and $19 billion in 1980.[2] The states are projected to spend $21.3 billion on Medicaid in fiscal 1987.

Premiums for private health insurance were about $100 billion in 1983, and about $77 billion of this cost was paid directly by employers; the remainder was paid by employees.[3] In addition, because many firms are now self-insured, their costs are not included in premium estimates. For each employee, the average annual health insurance contribution by employers amounted to $1,549 in 1984, or 7.4 percent of payroll.[4]

The increase in health care costs has consistently outpaced the growth of general prices. And although general price inflation explains a little over half of the steep increase in health care cost from the mid-1960s through the early 1980s, other factors within the health care sector have also been important.

Since 1970 there has been a rapid increase in demand for health care services, stimulated mainly by the growth of third-party financing. During the 1970s, the government paid an increasing share of health care expenditures for the elderly and the poor; private health insurance also expanded over this period.[5] In addition, because third-party payments made consumption increasingly unrelated to price, increased demand has placed strong upward pressure on prices. In effect, insurers reimbursed providers on the basis of their actual asking prices. This encouraged providers to raise prices and to increase the quantity of services per unit of treatment, and it favored the more costly or profitable services.

The rapid growth in government health care expenditures and the growth of private-sector employment-based benefits, in combination with reimbursement systems that exercised very little vigilance over providers' charges and practice patterns, made demand almost completely insensitive to price changes. Cost reimbursement transmitted a strong signal (and an open license) to providers to increase the use of labor and other resources. In addition, beginning in the late 1960s, the federal government provided enormous subsidies for medical education. The predictable result was a rapid increase in the number of health care professionals in excess of the growth in population. Between 1970 and 1980, some 23 new medical schools were established, the number of physicians per 100,000 population increased from 137 to 184, and the number of registered nurses per 100,000 population increased from 369 to 520.[6]

Providers shifted to more labor-intensive methods in the delivery of services. For example, the number of full-time equivalent employees per 100 average daily patients in community hospitals increased by 33 1/3 percent (from 302 to 402) between 1970 and 1981. This occurred at a time when there was virtually no increase in the number of community hospital beds per 1,000 population and a slight decline in occupancy rates. [7]

Employment has been growing more rapidly in the health care sector than in the rest of the economy. For example, in 1982, health care employment grew 4.3 percent as employment declined in the rest of the economy. The unemployment rate in the health care sector was less than half the national average. It is not surprising that as labor input expanded more rapidly than output, labor productivity growth in health care came to a virtual halt.

Sluggish productivity is one cause of the rapid increase in the real per capita cost of care provided. At the same time, the more intensive use of skilled labor undoubtedly increased the quality of care, which is difficult to capture in productivity statistics. Nevertheless, this more intensive use of labor and other inputs accounted for more than one-quarter of the increase in expenditures during the 1970s, with much of the source of this change attributable to expanding demand within a flawed reimbursement system. How to change that reimbursement system and achieve long-term gains in efficiency are the central policy issues facing public officials and private-sector decision makers.

POLICY TRENDS THAT CONTRIBUTE TO COST ESCALATION

Although some of the policy biases that generate cost escalation are most evident in government programs, they can also be found in private-sector policies.

FAULTY PAYMENT SYSTEMS

The dominant insurer in many regions of the country has been the Blue Cross, Blue Shield network of local organizations. When Blue Cross, Blue Shield was established a half century ago, physicians were deliberately included in the design of the system, and Blue Cross was clearly the dominant third-party payer. This led to a reimbursement system that did not distinguish among providers on the basis of the relative cost of their practice patterns or actual fees and charges. The concept of a "free choice of doctor," innocuous on its face, became a protection for providers against claims monitoring by the chief bill payers in the private sector. This was as true for commercial insurance carriers as for Blue Cross.

A lot has changed today. The Blue Cross, Blue Shield market share varies sharply from state to state, ranging from over 80 percent in Rhode Island to under 10 percent in Florida. Their average market share across the nation has fallen to 28 percent, as both the Blues and commercial insurers compete with the self-insurance option. In addition, many insurers have developed new cost discipline and preferred provider plans in an effort to remain viable.

The original Blue Cross model stressed front-end hospital coverage. The need for such coverage was apparent at the time because there was little insurance coverage for any health care services. In moving to meet this need, the insurance community established two patterns that have come back to haunt us: First, health coverage was tied to the *institution* (in this case the hospital), while preventive and primary services received much less attention. Second, health coverage was established on a *first-dollar* basis; that is, the *first* thirty days in a hospital were fully covered, but little or no coverage was provided for stays beyond this length. Thus, the problem of lack of catastrophic coverage was inherent in the early design of private health insurance. Private health insurance has also been skewed toward coverage for acute medical care and away from chronic care and care delivered in a home or community setting.

When Blue Cross and Blue Shield were first established, thirty-day hospital coverage was, as a practical matter, equivalent to catastrophic coverage because hospitalization was only for treating the very ill or for routine surgery. As hospitals gradually began providing routine care, the concept of first-dollar coverage made less and less economic sense and often failed to protect against unpredictable exposure to costly treatment involving more than routine care.

These built-in biases in private health insurance favoring institutional care, acute care designed in line with the medical model, and first-dollar coverage were copied in the design of Medicare and Medicaid. Not only was the cost payment system transported from the private to the public sector; so, too, were the basic boundaries of an insurance model that has led to serious imbalances in the types of services covered.

Traditionally, within the walls of a doctor's office, a hospital, or nursing home, an extra day of care, an extra test, an extra pill, and an extra bed have almost always been paid for by insurers, usually on a dollar-for-dollar basis. There have been a few exceptions (e.g., professional standards review organizations have questioned the length of some hospital stays for Medicare and Medicaid patients). But as a general rule, when health services are delivered inside a hospital or nursing home, they are paid for largely without question; and until recently, payment was on a cost-plus basis.

The basic flaws in both public- and private-sector payment systems may have served as a cushion for the introduction of higher-cost technology. Flawed payment systems insulate the purchasers of technology — in the first instance, hospitals, doctors, and other services providers, but ultimately those who pay their bills — from the need to make decisions about cost effectiveness. More important, innovations in drugs, equipment, and techniques that were cost-effective for diagnosing and treating specific conditions were often used unnecessarily, even if a less expensive technology was likely to be equally successful.

BIAS AGAINST PREVENTION AND OUTPATIENT CARE

Both government and private insurance programs have undervalued preventive care, chronic care, and care delivered in an outpatient or community setting at the same time that they have reimbursed costlier acute care provided in hospitals and doctors' offices. For example, Medicare legislation specifically differentiates between care in skilled nursing facilities and custodial care, allowing reimbursement for the former but not the latter. Indeed, in order to obtain coverage for treatment in a skilled nursing facility (which Medicare will cover up to a maximum of 100 days), a patient generally has to be certified as making progress toward a full recovery. Those lingering and not improving, particularly the aged, who arguably may be the most in need of financial assistance, may be excluded from coverage by such a criterion.

Medicare does not cover homemaker services or personal care services. Yet these are services that elderly persons may require in order to live at home, and their cost is likely to be much less than the cost of a nursing home. Medicare also does not pay for drugs or medicines that a patient purchases, with or without a prescription.

Outpatient treatment for mental illness is covered much less favorably than inpatient care. The maximum that Medicare can pay for outpatient psychiatric services, including rehabilitation, is $250 a year. In contrast, Medicare helps pay for up to 190 days (on a lifetime-maximum basis) of inpatient care.

Medicaid does permit states to cover preventive services, but wide variations in eligibility standards and covered services mean that such coverage depends very much on where the poor live. For example, a little over half of the states do not cover diagnostic, screening, or preventive care services.

In the private sector, some plans recognize the importance of prevention and the advantages of treatment in lower-cost institutional arrangements. Until recently, however, these plans have been exceptions. Most employer plans continue to be biased toward treatment of acute care for patients in higher-cost institutional settings.

RISING COST OF MALPRACTICE INSURANCE

The direct cost of malpractice insurance has been estimated at about $5 billion a year, or a little over 1 percent of total health care expenditures. But most observers believe that a more important source of costs related to malpractice involves so-called *defensive* medicine — that is, the extra tests and procedures, prolonged stays in hospitals, and more expensive technologies used by physicians to avoid being sued by patients. For example, there has been a sharp increase in Caesarean sections in recent years, and a greater use of such technologies as ultrasound and amniocentesis, and many experts attribute a large portion of this increase to precautions taken by obstetricians related to potential legal battles. There are also reports of obstetricians leaving the field to practice gynecology or other subspecialties that entail less risk of litigation.

IMPROVING ACCESS TO SERVICES

The federal government has directly increased the use of health care services by establishing insurance coverage for select groups — the elderly, a large segment of low-income households, veterans, and members of the armed services. Indirectly, it has increased the demand for services through the favorable tax treatment of employer contributions to employee health insurance and through making employee benefits a mandatory subject of collective bargaining.[8]

For many years during the postwar period, the federal government was also striving to expand the supply of health care personnel and facilities to assure that the growing demand was met. Through such measures as the Hill-Burton program encouraging hospital construction, federal grants to establish medical schools and support the tuition of medical students, and the huge investment in research funneled through the National Institutes of Health, the government added to the manpower, facilities, and knowledge base of the health care delivery system.

Over the past thirty years, employers and insurance carriers responded to public policy incentives to establish employer-based health insurance for workers and their families. In 1950, only about half of the civilian population was protected by one or more forms of private health insurance. By 1970, the protected population had risen to 78 percent; and by 1984, to 80 percent. Almost all those with health insurance are covered for inpatient hospital services. A large majority are also covered for outpatient diagnostic tests, mental health care, physician office visits, maternity care, and prescribed medicines. The rate of private insurance coverage for other health services is much lower. In 1977, 19 percent were covered for dental care, and only 8 percent were insured for vision and hearing care.[9] Since then, the total rate of coverage for these services has increased substantially; and for those covered under an employment-related group plan, the breadth of this coverage is now substantially higher.

Over the past two decades, the growth of private and public health insurance has enormously increased the access of almost all groups in society to medical care. In the 1960s, individuals earning less than $10,000 a year had on average fewer physician visits than higher-income groups. By 1976, income level had little effect on the number of visits per year; and by 1981, low-income groups had the highest number of visits. A complete convergence of visits per year has also occurred among patients of different races. And although patients in large metropolitan areas have slightly more visits per person than those living in other geographic areas, this difference has narrowed over time.[10]

REMAINING ACCESS PROBLEMS

Despite these benefits produced by the nation's increased investment in health care, there are groups whose access to medical care remains restricted because of lack of coverage through an employment-related health plan. Some are completely uninsured and are forced to forgo some needed care. When they do get care, this can impose indirect costs on others. In addition, uninsured persons are more likely to risk income losses through higher out-of-pocket expenses when they are ill.

The primary reason for the lack of health insurance is the inability of some workers to secure coverage during employment. Survey data indicate that uninsured employed workers and their dependents account for three-quarters of the 17 million persons who were uninsured during the 1977-1980 period.[11] A small proportion of unemployed workers (8 percent in 1977 and about 13 percent in 1982) lost health insurance as a result of unemployment. But these workers did not use less medical care in comparison with employed workers or with periods in which they were employed.[12]

Uninsured workers tend to be low-wage earners with low levels of education. Although a significant proportion of uninsured workers in 1977 were young adults aged nineteen to twenty-four and not firmly established in their careers, almost half were married and over thirty years of age. About 60 percent were full-time wage earners, and only about one-third were part-time workers.[13]

IMPROVING THE DISTRIBUTION OF INVESTMENT IN SERVICES

In attempting to provide health insurance protection for workers and their families, public policy has given workers and benefit managers incentives to develop employment-based programs. Individuals and employers responded to these incentives, accepting a larger proportion of their compensation in the form of insurance, the full value of which was excluded from taxable income. This expansion of health insurance protection was highly desirable.

Unfortunately, many employer plans initially adopted or moved toward first-dollar coverage, which, in combination with a payment system that frequently reimbursed providers fully on the basis of actual charges, encouraged some overconsumption of services. Employers were slow to recognize the connection between these features of their health care plans and escalating costs. In recent years, however, many employers have dropped first-dollar coverage and adopted various types of utilization reviews to reduce unnecessary consumption of services.

Public policy incentives also encouraged employers to extend coverage beyond hospitalization to include outpatient care and other major services. Protection against the high cost of services with a low probability of occurrence proved to be an extremely valuable form of insurance. In many cases, however, the incentives also encouraged benefit plan managers and employees to enrich plans by covering relatively low-cost routine services with a high probability of utilization, such as eyeglasses.

From the employer's perspective, including nonbasic services in health plans may be desirable, provided the payment system does not encourage unnecessary utilization or substantially raise the cost of premiums. From society's standpoint, however, if incentives to expand health insurance indirectly encourage overutilization of a wide range of services by some workers while other workers have no protection or are poorly protected against the costs of illness, an important issue is raised: how to design public policies that will improve the distribution of the nation's investment in health care. Both the private sector and the government are now faced with the challenge of designing policies that will discourage overutilization of services but at the same time protect those who lack access to affordable care.

IMPROVING THE QUALITY OF SERVICES

Health care quality is sometimes defined in terms of inputs into the system: the number of professionals per patient, the number of hospital beds per unit of the population, the availability of new medical procedures and drugs, and the type of training available to professionals. Despite the obvious weaknesses of using inputs to measure quality, the quality of care is likely to improve as inputs increase.*

By most of these measures, the U.S. health care system, on average, provides high-quality medical care; and the rising cost of inputs has produced significant benefits. Advances in medical science and the availability of new drugs to treat specific illnesses are evidence of increasing quality in the health care system, although it is more difficult to determine whether the benefits always exceed the costs of such quality improvements.

Quality improvements often involve a rather wholesale change in the nature of a service: new machines for diagnostic tests replace old ones, such as the substitution of nuclear magnetic resonance scanners for CAT scanners. New procedures quickly make yesterday's procedures obsolete. For example, cateract surgery is now performed either on an outpatient basis or with a very brief hospital stay; previously it required a seven- to ten-day hospital stay. A new product can reduce or eliminate the need for more expensive and risky procedures, as when new drugs have made exploratory surgery for ulcers unnecessary in many cases.

Most experts agree that the Medicaid system has had a positive effect on the health status of those low-income people who participate. The program has increased the access of the poor to health services to a level similar to the access available to the nonpoor.[14] A more specific example of the progress achieved in recent years is the significant decline in the death rate from major cardiovascular disease. Although a number of other developments undoubtedly contributed to this decline, it is likely that the government's Heart, Cancer, and Stroke Program, enacted in 1965, was a contributing factor.

Another indicator of success is the trend in infant mortality rates. Between 1965 and 1978, the death rate per 1,000 live births fell from 42 to 23 among blacks and from 22 to 12 among whites.[15] Relatively higher infant mortality rates for blacks persist, however, and are a source of continuing concern. Life expectancy at birth for males, which stood at 67.05 years in 1970, is estimated to reach 72.29 in 1990; for females, the figures are 74.80 in 1970 and 79.85 in 1990.[16] However, most of this improvement is probably due to better nutrition and healthier life-style behavior.

We have also seen dramatic breakthroughs in the treatment of disease as a result of new drugs. Penicillin and the polio vaccine are two notable examples. In recent years, there has been concern that the slowdown in the rate of innovation in the drug industry may have a detrimental effect on continued improvements in the quality of care.

It is important to avoid assuming that more care always translates into

---

*See memorandum by FRANKLIN A. LINDSAY (page 112).

better care. Indeed, there is evidence that when utilization among the insured population declines as a result of increased cost sharing or utilization controls imposed by HMOs, health status does not suffer noticeably.[17] The future quality of care provided by the U.S. health care system depends as much on how the investment is made as on the magnitude of the expenditures.

Assessing the quality of care will always involve subjective judgment. What is needed in an effective health care system is assurance that patients are guided toward providers who meet acceptable standards of performance. Greater effort must be made by the private and public sectors to develop criteria for judging quality.

BALANCING COST CONTAINMENT WITH IMPROVED ACCESS AND QUALITY OF CARE

In the past several years, actions by the government and industry have reduced the rate of increase in health care costs although the rate remains higher than the increase for consumer prices generally. Clearly, then, the cost problem has not been solved. Demographic trends indicate that upward pressure on the demand for services will continue, especially from older Americans, who proportionately are health care's highest consumers.

In 1980, the median age of the U.S. population was thirty years; but by 2010, it is expected to be thirty-eight years.[18] The proportion of the population age sixty-five and over will continue to grow throughout the remainder of this century and escalate rapidly once the baby boom generation reaches retirement age. Pressure to expand costly long-term care services for the elderly will escalate as a larger proportion of the elderly (those sixty-five and over) reach seventy-five, an age when the probability of requiring long-term care increases sharply. In 1980, about 39 percent of the elderly were seventy-five or over; by 2000, the proportion will have soared to 49 percent.

Over the next twenty years, as the large group of World War II and Korean veterans age, government expenditures for health care services for elderly veterans are likely to increase significantly. Under current policy, once veterans reach sixty-five, they are entitled to health care at minimum cost, even if an illness is not service-related.

Actions to constrain cost increases will also have to take into account the need to maintain quality and improve access. It is unacceptable politically to keep costs down by further reducing the access of low-income workers to services and at the same time expect the working population to pay much of the cost of care for the elderly. Such a strategy makes no economic sense because any money saved by reducing the access of low-income workers will be offset by an increase in the cost of indigent care. Similarly, it is unacceptable to lower costs by cutting back significantly on the quality of care.

Society will benefit from policies that ensure equality between the overall benefits and expenditures. Given the large geographic variations in the expenditures necessary for similar procedures and treatment goals and the fact that lower-cost services often do not appear to reduce quality of care, there appears to be considerable scope for achieving the societal goals of cost containment, assured access, and high quality of care by reallocating resources to those services and individuals who will benefit most. Thus, it may be possible to achieve these goals without increasing the proportion of GNP invested in health care.

However, it would be misleading to suggest that government and private-sector actions which redistribute resources to increase the overall benefit from health care expenditures will not reduce the access and quality of care now available to *some* individuals. Because individuals pay less than the market price for services, some additional consumption of care provides benefits that exceed the cost to the individual, but do not exceed the social costs of providing that care. The benefit to society of providing low-income workers and their families with better access to care is likely to be greater than subsidizing additional care for the nonpoor elderly, but many elderly individuals will not view it that way.

We believe that it should be possible to develop a health care policy that reduces cost escalation and continues to improve quality without necessarily reducing access for those least able to afford services. Much can be done to improve the management of health care delivery and to increase efficiency through innovation. It is also possible to achieve some savings by reducing the cost of inputs to the production of health services. In the final analysis, however, if the nation is to achieve the goals of cost constraint, improved access, and high quality simultaneously, both public- and private-sector policies will have to be modified to reduce the consumption of services by some groups in society.

Chapter 3

Government Involvement and Incentives in Health Care Markets

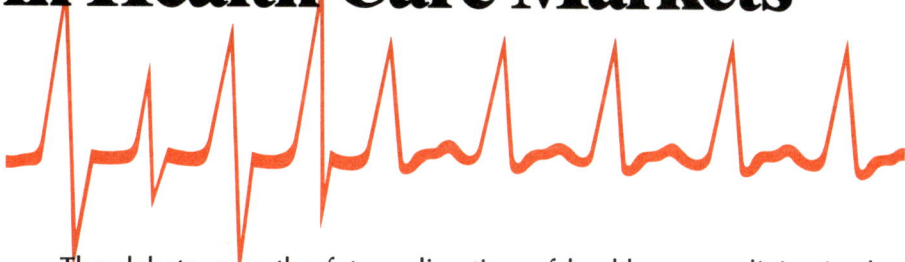

The debate over the future direction of health care policies in the United States is not over the legitimacy of government's responsibility to influence the demand for and supply of services. Rather, it is about whether the continuous growth of government intervention in markets has stimulated or retarded the quest for cost control, innovation, and increased access to services.

Government is involved in the U.S. health care system in a variety of ways. In some cases the government provides services directly, as in programs for military personnel and veterans. The consumption of care is heavily subsidized for some groups, such as the elderly and the poor. For the working population, there is preferential treatment of employer contributions to health insurance benefits. In some markets, production has been heavily subsidized, as in the case of the education and training of health care professionals. In other instances, the government only influences the environment in which large numbers of firms compete actively for market share. For example, in many supplier markets such as pharmaceuticals, government regulation is intended only to protect consumers against potential adverse effects of new products.

States regulate the insurance industry. But insurance companies, which play a key role in administration and design of employer health plans, still compete actively in the market for group insurance with each other and with large employers, who often decide to self-insure their employees against the risk of illness. The hospital market is dominated by nonprofit institutions that receive tax advantages from federal, state, and local governments. Private nonprofit organizations represent more than half of all community hospitals, and state and local government hospitals account for 29 percent. Investor-owned hospitals account for only 14 percent of community hospitals, but their number has been growing in recent years.

The distinction among the different forms of community hospitals is diminishing. It is difficult to distinguish between the markets served by the for-profit and nongovernment nonprofit hospitals. Both appear to serve about the same proportion of patients who cannot or refuse to pay for services (3 to 5 percent of patient revenues).[1] However, state and local government hospitals remain somewhat unique and are more likely to be located in areas with a larger proportion of the underinsured population. As a result, their combined bad debts and charity costs are about 10 to 12 percent of their gross patient revenues.

THE ROLE OF THE MARKET SYSTEM

In markets for most products and services, economic efficiency is enhanced if government intervention is minimal and competition thrives. Efficiency is achieved through the strong incentive for suppliers to minimize costs and respond to demand by allocating resources to their most productive uses. The market also enhances the goal of innovation by providing powerful incentives for management to surpass both its own past performance and that of its competitors. But private-sector markets do not always achieve the desired results; outcomes may be socially unacceptable. In health care, this is especially important because some reasonable minimum level of access for everyone is as important as the goals of good cost management and a high rate of innovation.

Incentives for efficiency and innovation are frequently absent in many health care markets. For market incentives to produce efficiency and innovation, buyers must be aware of the range of prices for similar packages of coverage for medical treatment and must be motivated to accept the lowest price for care of a particular quality. This requires that purchasers have the ability to judge the quality of service available and make a choice based on price differences. It also presupposes that there are a sufficient number of suppliers of the service who are actively competing to provide it and that there are a substantial number of individuals or institutions deciding what type of service to consume.

Competitive conditions vary among health care markets. For example, the market for hospital services is dominated by nonprofit institutions that often have fewer incentives to minimize cost through efficiency and innovation than for-profit institutions do. Available evidence suggests, however, that the profit motive does not appear to result in any significant difference between the care provided to patients and the cost efficiency for either type of institution.[2] At the other extreme, the production of new drugs and medical equipment is provided almost entirely by for-profit businesses. These private-sector organizations continuously search for profitable opportunities through the expansion of market share and the development of new products in response to consumer demand for more effective treatment.

The extreme complexity of many health care procedures makes it difficult for the consumer to act as an informed buyer. Consequently, when individuals seek treatment for life-threatening or even routine illnesses, they are unlikely to respond to differences in price. In most cases, however, given sufficient information on quality and prices, consumer behavior, in the absence of government intervention, is likely to be responsive to price differences. Moreover, it is in the selection of an insurance plan, usually once a year, that consumers should be most cognizant of comparative costs.

In the markets for physicians' services and hospital care, the individual's personal physician, hospital, or employer often selects the service provider. This obscures the individual's knowledge of prices and quality, and it complicates the precise nature of the demand for the service since each participant in the decision has a different interest in the cost and benefits arising from the choice of treatment.

In the past, most employers and their insurance carriers failed to increase consumer choice and to encourage the cost-conscious use of health care services by employees. Until recently, the private sector has also failed to come to grips with the problem of rising cost of employee health insurance.

The fact that the U.S. health care system is dominated by employment-based health plans provides employers with a unique opportunity to overcome the lack of information individuals have about the services offered. The specialized experience of health plan benefit managers and those designing plans in the insurance industry can significantly increase consumer and employer information about the range of prices and quality of services available. We believe employers can both give employees protection against illness and at the same time provide incentives for providers to compete for a share of the demand for services.

While there are obvious limitations on the extent to which market principles can be expected to achieve the goals of health care policies, government intervention also has serious limitations. Indeed, in some cases the growth of the government role is actually the primary cause of the failure of private markets.

Extensive government intervention in the market for hospital services through Medicare illustrates how public policy can contribute to market failure. Although hospitals have no strong incentive to minimize cost, they do compete with other institutions that can offer alternative services. Consequently, nonprofit hospitals attempt to increase the number of patients they serve by offering an extensive range of diagnostic and therapeutic services in order to encourage more physicians to recommend their patients.

The cost-reimbursement system of the Medicare regulations (prior to the introduction of the DRG payment system) and the relative importance of Medicare payments to hospital revenues, in combination with the unusual incentives facing nonprofit institutions, made it much more difficult to contain escalating costs.

HOW GOVERNMENT INTERVENES

There are essentially two competing strategies for controlling health care cost escalation, increasing innovation, and improving access: one is to increase government regulation, or at least strengthen and improve the effectiveness of existing regulations; the other is to reduce government regulations and use market incentives to change the behavior of the participants in health care markets.

An extreme form of regulation would involve the indirect public provision of health care through some form of national health insurance (NHI). The types of national health plans proposed in the 1970s linked extensions of coverage to the uninsured with a complex national budgeting system designed to squeeze the private health care sector. Indeed, successive versions of these national health proposals carried relatively lower federal price tags but increasingly complex regulatory schemes for private insurance. In effect, the cost was moved, in part, out of government budgets and into private-sector budgets (e.g., mandates that employers must provide comprehensive coverage to all employees). These proposals advocated paying for greater coverage by holding down doctors' fees through negotiations between the government and physicians and by establishing rigid multilayered local, state, and national budgets for hospital expenditures.

In contrast, more recent proposals, such as the Consumer Choice Health Plan developed by Alain C. Enthoven, would rely on a system of capped refundable federal income tax credits to achieve both universal access to care and a more competitive, less regulated private sector. The Enthoven plan would rely on a voucher-type approach to subsidizing low-income people that separates eligibility for health care subsidies from the arbitrary categorical restrictions built into the current welfare system. It rejects paying for such subsidies through regulatory controls on the private sector.

Under the regulatory NHI plans, universal coverage would be phased in through an expansion of the Medicare-Medicaid program to include access to care for all individuals. Even under the more off-budget versions, public expenditures for health care would increase substantially. The current system of employment-based health insurance could be retained, but the government would regulate these plans, and the method of paying providers would be changed. The major advantage claimed for this approach is that it would guarantee adequate health care for all and that for individuals with no insurance or insufficient insurance, it would remove the threat of financial ruin from health care bills. However, experience shows that despite the increase in access, consumption of care still varies with income. This is because higher-income groups have a greater incentive to invest in health care even within a highly regulated system.[3]

There is no doubt that this type of regulatory approach would improve the certainty that all individuals would have access to services. But its contribution to the goal of improved quality of care is much more doubtful. This extreme form of regulatory control also seriously fails to contribute to the goal of the efficient allocation of resources. Under extensive government regulation, there is no automatic mechanism to ensure that resources are allocated efficiently, and there is substantial evidence indicating that attempts by government to regulate the distribution of resources reduces efficiency.[4]

REGULATION OF INSURANCE

Insurance regulations are designed to assure the financial solvency of health insurance plans so that policyholders are not vulnerable to sudden loss of coverage. Unfortunately, the application of these regulations often acts as a barrier to competition.

A number of insurance regulations at the federal and state levels seem to favor companies that self-insure (a rapidly growing development) over those insured by insurance companies, particularly commercial ones. The Employee Retirement Income Security Act (ERISA) exempts self-insured companies from state regulation of health insurance.

For those insurers who are regulated by state commissioners, several aspects of regulation are cause for concern. For example, reserve requirements tie up funds of employers insured by either Blue Cross or commercial carriers; to the extent that such funds exceed the amount of reserves employers would set aside on their own, they reflect forgone interest that self-insuring companies do not have to incur. Self-insurers are also not subject to investment regulations, (e.g., that no more than a specified percentage of assets be invested in common stocks, corporate bonds, or debentures). Initial solvency requirements are often lower for Blue Cross, Blue Shield than for commercial insurers, and the Blues are exempt from state premium taxes that commercial insurers must pay.

In addition, many states have imposed benefit requirements on the commercials and the Blues that self-insurers are not obligated to honor. Over the past decade, there has been a tenfold increase in mandated benefit laws, from roughly 50 to over 600 at the end of 1985. Services required by such laws include treatment for alcohol and drug abuse, psychology, optometry, chiropractors' services, nurse midwives, and in vitro fertilization.

Such requirements can be a barrier to a competitive environment because they rule out the ability to offer consumers and employers varying combinations of coverage and cost. Some consumers, for example, may prefer an insurance package that offers a full line of benefits for hospital coverage, doctors' visits, X rays, and laboratory tests but excludes treatment by a chiropractor or psychologist. Other consumers might prefer the more comprehensive package that costs a little more but removes the risk of exposure to higher outlays for more services. A broad system of mandated benefits precludes this type of decision making. It could lead to national health insurance through the back door, and it could encourage smaller employers to drop coverage altogether.

REGULATION OF MARKET ENTRY

In a similar fashion, state occupational licensing laws and scope-of-practice limitations constrict the choices available to patients. Of course, licensing is necessary to assure a minimum level of training and competence, but a valid regulatory activity can be taken too far in the name of consumer protection. Such regulation can be used for another purpose that has little to do with the consumer protection banner under which it flies: the protection of the earnings levels to which certain health professionals have become accustomed. New types of professional specialties such as nurse practitioner or psychiatric social worker are maturing and trying to obtain a foothold in the market. Measures such as scope-of-practice limitations can restrict the ability of these professionals to compete effectively with more traditional health care providers.

So-called freedom-of-choice and antidiscrimination laws imposed by states prohibit insurers from encouraging subscribers to select lower-cost providers by paying a higher percentage of the bills of relatively lower costs. The very names applied to these laws make it difficult to argue with their purpose. But if insurers are proscribed from distinguishing between relatively more cost-effective providers and those deemed to practice overly elaborate or expensive medicine, the essence of a competitive market for insurance is lost.

Extensive government regulation makes it extremely difficult to measure changes in the relative prices of services. This leads to continuous shortages and surpluses in health care markets, with government planners constantly trying to adjust prices. Extensive regulation also provides few incentives to minimize costs. In response, price controls to contain inflation are often advocated and have sometimes been adopted. In the short run, this distorts the allocation of resources, and in the long run, such controls seriously discourage innovation and make it necessary to ration access to care and/or reduce the quality of services.

CONTROLLING SUPPLY TO HOLD DOWN COSTS

Since the mid-1970s, public policy has tried to control costs by controlling the supply of health care facilities. The government required hospitals to have prior approval for adding new facilities through a certificate-of-need process, a right granted by a local health services agency that allows construction, expansion, or modernization of health care facilities.

This program has had only a marginal effect (if any) on the supply of hospital facilities, partially because it covered only a small proportion of the overall inefficiencies that contribute to cost escalation and partially because the local planning apparatus has often fallen victim to efforts to evade or circumvent the regulatory process. Even if the certificate-of-need process were successful in completing the difficult task of determining the precise number and size of hospital facilities that meet the local community's needs at the lowest cost, it might simply encourage cost escalation in some other part of the system for delivery of institutional care. For example, it might encourage more extensive use of existing services simply to justify additional facilities. Or it might make it more difficult for alternative forms of institutional care to enter the market and compete with traditional hospitals.

Other efforts have focused on how hospitals will be reimbursed for services. Many of these complex state rate-setting approaches have tried to build in incentives for hospitals to reduce the average length of stay. One of the drawbacks of regulating the price of hospital services is that it addresses only the symptoms of the problem. A major reason for the cost escalation is that the delivery system contains no incentives to constrain increases in the intensity and rate of utilization of care. Consequently, control of rate setting has apparently had only a modest effect on lowering costs and increasing the efficiency of service delivery.

Those states that have introduced compulsory prospective reimbursement programs seem to have been somewhat more successful in slowing the rate of cost escalation than states that have no such program.[5] This was one of the factors that encouraged the Reagan Administration to introduce the prospective rate-setting approach embodied in the DRG reform of the Medicare program.

To the extent that providers incur large deficits as a consequence of rate regulation, public officials must be prepared to permit inefficient suppliers to fail and go out of business. Experience shows that public officials have avoided making these difficult decisions. More important, rate regulation may produce some short-term slowing of cost escalation; but in the long run, it is likely to create significant market distortions thereby producing an inefficient distribution of resources.

TOWARD GREATER RELIANCE ON MARKET INCENTIVES

It is essential that consumers have the opportunity to make choices among types of service and that their decisions to some extent affect their personal finances. This raises the difficult issue of the extent to which individuals should pay part of their medical care cost under both government programs such as Medicare and private employment-based health insurance plans.

If a third party pays the full cost of care, with no direct contribution from the individual, consumers are unresponsive to price and quality differences and tend to select the most expensive care and most desirable amenities.

Traditional insurance plans did not provide incentives for patients to choose efficient over inefficient providers. In part, this type of insurance developed because tax incentives encouraged employers to provide part of their employees' compensation in the form of payment of health care insurance premiums that were not included in the employees' taxable incomes. This tax incentive has produced substantial benefits to a very high proportion of the population. It has also produced public benefits by greatly reducing the need for society to pay the health care costs for individuals who have no insurance.

Full insurance protection against any individual cost destroys the market's ability to allocate health resources efficiently. But if individuals have no insurance and cannot pay the full cost of treatment, the cost of providing uncompensated care is shifted to the rest of society. Also, uninsured people often neglect their health and do not seek some needed health services that could prevent more serious, high-cost illnesses later. The goal of introducing demand-side market incentives into employment-based insurance plans is to strike a balance between 100 percent insurance against all costs of illness on one hand and the opposite extreme of large unpaid bills when the individual has no insurance or insurance that pays only a small proportion of the actual cost.

One way to reach a compromise is for the health insurance contract to require the individual to pay a proportion of the cost of the treatment, perhaps 20 percent. This *coinsurance* (the proportion paid by the individual) encourages the individual to consider alternative forms of care based on costs.

Making the individual responsible for part of the cost requires providers to compete on the basis of cost as well as quality of care and amenities. In order to maintain or increase their share of the market, providers must try to avoid raising prices and must improve the efficiency of services. If there is significant competition, providers may have to lower prices to ensure demand for their services.

Insurance companies, often in cooperation with benefit managers for employment-based plans, can also play an important role in stimulating price and quality competition among providers. This can be done by monitoring claims and negotiating lower payments for claims thought to be excessive. Requiring prior approval for nonemergency surgery and second surgical opinions also introduces market incentives.

A combination of more reliance on market incentives and more explicit recognition of government's role in health care markets is the type of strategy most likely to achieve the health care policy goals of cost restraint and increased innovation and, at the same time, improve government policies to ensure access to a reasonable level of medical care for all. Government should continue to intervene in health care markets whenever private markets cannot do the job. Throughout the remainder of this policy statement, proposals for improvements in both public and private health care policies are presented. The principal theme underlying these proposals is that market-type incentives have a central role in the reform of all health care policies in the public as well as the private sector.

Chapter 4

Market Incentives and Employer Innovations

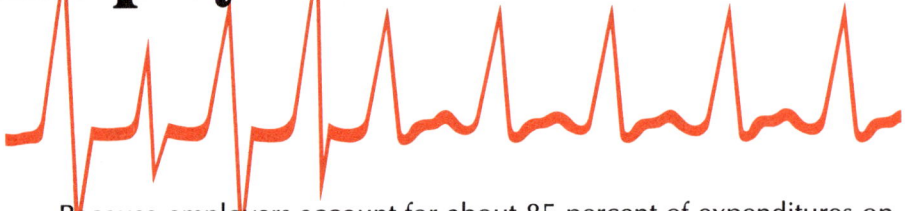

Because employers account for about 85 percent of expenditures on employment-based health care insurance, they are in a crucial position to affect the design of market incentives. CED believes that employers should use this opportunity to improve market incentives through private-sector policies.

Employers can take several types of steps to help reduce health costs: improving workplace safety, stimulating employee participation in health improvement programs, redesigning health benefits, and collecting data on the charges and practice patterns of health care providers.

IMPROVING WORKPLACE SAFETY

An effective prevention strategy is likely to have an extremely high pay-off for employers and employees in terms of reduced health care costs and absenteeism because of illness. One of the most effective ways to reduce employer costs is to develop programs that minimize employee exposure to known hazards. The government has an important role in reducing work-place hazards through safety regulations, but because managers and employees involved in the actual production of goods and services usually have better information, it is essential that management enforce its own safety rules.

- **CED recommends that top-level managers make effective safety programs for prevention of accidents and exposure to hazardous substances a corporate goal. The standards of health and safety should be based on best practices within the industry and, wherever possible, should exceed standards mandated by government regulation.**

In many industries, job performance in certain occupations can affect the health and safety of workers and the general public. Drug abuse by employees in these occupations is likely to harm others and increase a business's liability risks. CED therefore believes that all employers in industries where this exists should, within the limits prescribed by law, consider introducing a drug testing program for employees.

Although rehabilitation is not possible for all injuries, an effective program should be an integral part of the employer's health care policy and the initial phase of a strategy for reducing the cost of accidents.[1] When rehabilitation is appropriate, the combination of early intervention with second opinions on diagnosis of injury and a monitoring system for proposed treatment is vital to reducing the cost of injuries to both employers and employees.

STIMULATING EMPLOYEE PARTICIPATION IN HEALTH IMPROVEMENT PROGRAMS

Educational programs directed at drug and alcohol abuse, safety programs aimed at reducing accidents and preventing exposure to hazardous substances, and fitness programs involving weight control and exercise can provide real benefits to companies seeking to lower health care costs.

More than one-third of the 100 companies that responded to a CED survey have some type of formal health promotion program for their employees.[2] Many knowledgeable company officials are quick to note that wellness programs may not necessarily translate directly or quickly into lower health care costs. In the short run, such programs may do more to raise employee morale and reduce absenteeism than to improve health. Of course, improved employee morale and attendance can enhance productivity, which will reduce unit production costs and improve the competitiveness of the enterprise.

Effective wellness programs clearly need to incorporate evaluation procedures and cannot be viewed as a panacea for all health issues. Nevertheless, these programs can be cost effective and, on average, can improve health and prolong life. Johnson & Johnson's Live for Life program (see page 36) demonstrates the strengths of such programs.

- **CED recommends that all employers adopt wellness programs as part of company health care policy.**

Voluntary participation in wellness programs should be encouraged, and employers may want to consider economic incentives to heighten employee interest. Many types of behavior, such as smoking, drug use, and excessive consumption of alcohol, are likely to have an adverse effect on health. But since the harm these substances cause varies with each individual, there is little justification for penalizing behavior which imposes no cost on our fellow employees or society in general. If, however, the lifestyle and behavior of some employees impose costs on fellow workers, or adversely affect work performance, employers are justified in penalizing

AN EMPLOYEE WELLNESS PROGRAM AS THE FOUNDATION OF COST CONTROL STRATEGY: JOHNSON & JOHNSON'S LIVE FOR LIFE PROGRAM

The Live for Life program is the central component of Johnson & Johnson's strategy to hold down the illness costs of employees and their families. The other components include benefits design (e.g. deductibles), workplace safety efforts, and the application of traditional occupational medicine at the work site.

The program's goal is to promote better employee health by achieving specific improvements in nutrition, weight control, physical fitness, cessation of smoking, management of stress and monitoring of blood pressure. The program is voluntary, so management makes a major marketing effort to enroll employees.

Top management has committed financial resources, made the program a managerial responsibility throughout the company, and responded to employee requests for improvements in the work environment. The program is launched by a volunteer committee drawn from top and middle managers and labor leaders. The goal is to enroll 80 percent of employees in the initial phase.

There are four main components of the Live for Life Program: In the initial phase, employees are offered the opportunity to receive an assessment of their current health status through a Health Screen. This phase is followed by the Lifestyle Seminar, a series of three-hour seminars for groups of fifty employees.

The Live for Life staff is responsible for conducting the Lifestyle Seminar and ensuring that each employee who participates in the Health Screen receives a lifestyle profile. Company leaders are primarily responsible for the promotion, recruitment, and scheduling of employees into the Lifestyle Seminar. They are also responsible for presenting to employees the health enhancement opportunities available through the program during the coming year. A target of 75 percent employee participation is the goal for this phase.

The third component is the Action Programs for lifestyle improvement. Action Programs are offered regularly in smoking cessation, weight control, that type of behavior. Recognizing the difficulties of defining unhealthy lifestyles and behavior, CED recommends that employers, along with insurance carriers, experiment with the development of a system of economic incentives and penalties, including differential health insurance rates, which encourage employees to engage in healthy lifestyles.

Employers should also consider attempting to "individualize" informa-

---

stress management, nutrition, exercise, and high blood pressure control. They use a variety of formats, including groups, individual consultation, self-help kits, and the telephone. In addition, Live for Life regularly offers a wide range of shorter educational and promotional programs built on such topics as breast self-examination, biofeedback, nutrition, and blood pressure.

The Live for Life staff is responsible for making sure that the programs are carefully tested and that trained professionals conduct them. Moreover, the staff conducts ongoing audits to ensure that all lifestyle improvement programs meet professional quality and performance standards. A report on the quality and performance of all these programs is supplied by the staff to company leaders regularly.

The fourth component consists of programs to sustain participation in the Action Programs. Employees are given noneconomic incentives, such as small gifts, for success in meeting a numerical health improvement goal. The staff also conducts follow-up phone and mail inquiries asking those who have participated in the seminars to report their improvements in weight loss, smoking cessation, and so on.

Key to the Live for Life strategy is a continuous effort to measure the success of the program through an independent evaluation. The measurements are based on a comparison of performances of the participants in Live for Life with a control group of nonparticipants for the years 1979 through 1983. The program has demonstrated that it contributes to profitability. Over the first two years of the program, participants showed a significant decline (15 percent) in lost working time because of illness, compared with the much poorer performance (a 3 percent increase) of those employees in a control group. Wellness strategies can not only be popular benefits programs but, if properly executed, can also contribute to the long-run efficiency of the enterprise. The program initially involved a net additional cost to the business. Within a few years, however, there was a significant reduction in the cost of hospitalization per employee that clearly justifies the start-up investment. For an employee who did not participate in Live for Life, Johnson & Johnson spent $104 in 1979 in hospital dollars. That amount increased to $465 by 1983. In comparison, for those with Live for Life, the company spent $100 for each employee in 1979 and $324 in 1983.

tion for health improvement. On the basis of traits and genetic characteristics, individuals have different probabilities of developing health problems such as heart disease, stroke, and excessive weight. These probabilities depend on the individual's own physical characteristics as well as his lifestyle. Employers should encourage their employees to participate in health assessment programs which make individuals aware of the kind of lifestyle most appropriate to their own health profile. In this case, however, any information on individual traits or genetic characteristics should be completely confidential to the individual and to the physician making the assessment and recommending the appropriate behavior.

COLLECTING DATA ON PROVIDER CHARGES AND PRACTICE PATTERNS

Another key ingredient in the recipe for a competitive market is the collection, analysis, and use of data on charges and practice patterns of health care providers. Some large corporations, such as American Telephone & Telegraph Co. (see page 39), have developed data systems that form provider profiles. These profiles permit comparisons of the different providers serving employees in a community and enable the purchasers of health services to identify those doctors or hospitals whose charges appear out of line with community norms. Honeywell Inc. is working with the Mayo Clinic to develop comparative utilization profiles for comparable populations as a tool for use with providers who serve its employees.

A number of health care coalitions around the country have been active in developing provider profiles. For example, the Midwest Business Group on Health (MBGH) has developed a model format for the presentation of claims data, and several major commercial insurance companies and Blue Cross have adopted it for providing data to their customers. A good reporting system that permits meaningful comparisons requires a uniform data set, and MBGH has developed specifications for a minimum set of data elements for claims processing. Currently, about two-thirds of MBGH's 120 member companies are organized into ten user groups to share claims data that, on a pooled basis, permits the detection of areawide patterns of service use and costs.

The Health Policy Corporation of Iowa is also serving a large group of employers by organizing a unified data base that facilitates the construction of provider profiles. Increasingly, companies are working with coalitions of insurers and providers to make quality of health care as important a goal as cost containment. Pennsylvania's Buy Right Strategy (see page 40) illustrates the type of private-sector action now emerging in many areas.

A MEDICAL EXPENSE PLAN DATA BASE: AMERICAN TELEPHONE & TELEGRAPH CO.

American Telephone & Telegraph Co. (AT&T) currently covers some 1.2 million people (active and retired employees and their dependents) under its Medical Expense Plans, with projected costs around $790 million in 1986. Because of the dollar magnitude, medical expenses have been an ongoing concern in the management of corporate resources.

During the early 1970s, the cost of maintaining health insurance grew at the rate of about 20 percent a year. As a result, the company in 1977 incorporated various cost- and quality-control measures, including voluntary second surgical opinion, preadmission testing, coverage for ambulatory surgical facilities and outpatient treatment, and an increasing company contribution to HMOs. These measures helped, and the rate of increase in costs moderated. Between 1980 and 1983, however, health care costs again began to accelerate, at an average annual rate of 22 percent. To obtain a better understanding of plan usage, the company in 1981 began development of its Medical Expense Plan data base. This data base includes all the information about claims that AT&T's insurance carriers, as claims payers, collect. Claims are then processed to create episodic records; that is, all claims relating to an episode of illness (hospital, laboratory, surgeons' fees, related physician visits, and so on) are grouped together. Such data help to measure the effectiveness of cost containment activities, serve as inputs for future plan design, and are used to evaluate the patterns and quality of medical care.

In 1983, additional plan changes redirected utilization toward less costly outpatient settings. A number of cost-containment programs were developed for implementation during 1986 and 1987. To coordinate and facilitate these activities, a corporate medical cost manager was appointed in April 1985.

AT&T's major cost-containment effort is the Medical Utilization Review Program. Its features include hospital preadmission certification, mandatory second surgical opinion, concurrent review, individual case management, expanded alternative care facilities, and enhanced health care information services for employees. In support of this, a major employee education program has been conducted, and an integrated health awareness/wellness program may be added. It is anticipated that these activities will have a significant positive impact, limiting the increase in costs, promoting an associated sentinel effect, and generally improving the nature and quality of health care.

CED believes that business organizations should encourage the establishment of information clearing houses based on the models developed by existing business health care coalitions. Moreover, although information is most effectively delivered at the local and regional levels, it should be possible for the regional offices of the federal government to assist in the development of this type of information system.

IMPROVING CONSUMER CHOICE

The ability of consumers to choose among different suppliers of services can be a powerful incentive for the market system to stimulate innovations and provide services efficiently. Before the 1980s, employees had very little choice of private-sector health care plans. A 1977 government

PENNSYLVANIA BUY RIGHT STRATEGY

In order to "buy right," companies must be prepared to change fundamentally the way they currently purchase health care and, thus, avoid premium increases which have averaged more than 9 percent annually for the past five years. The general steps a company can take are outlined below.

First, companies must identify low-cost, high-quality providers. Firms can move to request that their insurer supply this information. Within local areas, companies can work together and with providers to produce price and quality data.

For insured and self-insured firms, several business health coalitions in Pennsylvania are now developing the necessary information for their members, using the Pennsylvania Business Roundtable's Claims Pooling, Analysis, and Reporting System (CPARS). In addition, business, union, and health industry leaders are seeking to create a statewide health price and quality data system, to be made available to the public. This system could produce results by late 1987.

Second, companies must initiate a health care cost reduction educational program for their employees. There are many models of successful programs of this kind now under way, including Air Products & Chemicals in Allentown; Sun Company in Philadelphia; Alcoa in Pittsburgh; and the Lord Corporation in Erie. Local business/health coalitions can help design such programs for members, and the Pennsylvania Business Roundtable will provide background materials. Employees need to understand how they can make a difference in controlling costs, how they can improve their health and that of their families, and how the "buy right" program works.

survey of 10,000 households found that 82 percent of employees receiving health insurance through the workplace had no choice of health plan — only one was offered. Where choices did exist, they were typically biased in favor of the higher-cost plans; employers typically paid either the full cost of all plans or a constant *proportion* of the premiums of the various plans instead of a fixed-dollar amount.[3] An equally reliable up-to-date measure of the incidence and nature of plan choice is not available, but the 1987 edition of the National Medical Care Expenditure Survey (which was first conducted in 1977) should show a sharp gain in the availability of choice.

More choice in employee group health insurance has been stimulated by the federal requirement that firms employing twenty-five or more workers offer a federally qualified HMO to their employees if one is available in their market area. This dual-choice requirement has been in force since the early-1970s, and although it probably led many firms to *offer* HMOs, it is

---

The first and most essential step is the acquisition of information. The text of any company's health care arrangement should be: Does this plan provide employees with excellent care at the lowest comparative cost among providers? If so, it fits the "buy right" strategy.

On the basis of the "buy right" approach, pioneered by Walter McClure and the Center for Policy Studies, the Pennsylvania Business Roundtable has adopted the "Pennsylvania Buy Right Strategy" as the method by which purchasers and consumers of care, companies and their employees, can significantly reduce health care costs and eliminate many of the cost-inflating economic incentives which characterize the current system of medical care. The key to lower health care costs — while maintaining quality and access — is for all purchasers to purchase care based on its quality and price. Overall costs can be reduced by 20 to 30 percent without affecting quality. This amounts to potential annual savings of as much as $500 per employee at today's costs, without reducing benefits.

Many of the leaders of the health care delivery and financing industries in Pennsylvania agree that the "buy right" strategy makes sense for Pennsylvanians. The Hospital Association of Pennsylvania, Pennsylvania Blue Shield, Pennsylvania Association of Health Maintenance Organizations, Blue Cross of Western Pennsylvania, Capital Blue Cross, Blue Cross of Northeastern Pennsylvania, and the Pennsylvania Medical Society have joined with the Roundtable and Pew Memorial Trust to carry out a three-year educational program in major health care markets to implement the "buy right" strategy in a responsible and effective manner.

SOURCE: Pennsylvania Business Roundtable, *The Pennsylvania Buy Right Strategy for Medical Care* (Harrisburg, Penn., 1986).

only more recently that employees are *selecting* HMOs in significantly larger numbers. Indeed, HMO enrollment reached 26.7 million in December 1984, or about 7 percent of the U.S. population, a 22 percent increase over December 1983.[4] Consumer choice has been expanded through the recent growth in preferred provider organizations (PPOs) with more than 300 now in existence throughout the country.

The growth of PPOs may actually prove to be more significant than the growth of HMOs. These PPO plans typically include both selected (preferred) and nonselected (nonpreferred) providers, with cost-sharing differentials applicable at point of use. In other words, if a beneficiary in a PPO selects a preferred provider, cost sharing is either lowered or completely waived. Providers can be considered preferred not only on the basis of fees and charges per unit of services but also on the basis of their history of hospital admissions, length of stay, number of tests and procedures, and other uses of resources. PPOs offer the physicians and hospitals such benefits as prompt payment and assured volume of patients in return for price moderation.

PPOs provide the type of incentives to hold down costs found in HMOs, while retaining the basic elements of freedom to choose among a broad array of providers in a community. Employees who choose the PPO option are free to select nonpreferred providers but will pay a little extra if they do. This creates an incentive, but not an absolute mandate, for consumers to obtain health care services from preferred providers. PPOs rely on utilization reviews and negotiated fee schedules to put pressure on providers, but in return typically promise prompt payment and settlement of claims.

A key ingredient in the recipe for a competitive market is the practice of equal payments by employers to the various plans offered. A fixed-dollar contribution in a given year (which could be updated each year) could be pegged at the level of the most cost-effective plan being offered. Employees selecting a higher-cost plan would have to add some of their own money to cover the relatively higher cost of the premium. In 1983, Wisconsin adopted this approach for state employees, pegging its fixed contribution at the average cost of HMOs. In the first open enrollment period following this change, there was a dramatic increase in the proportion of state workers choosing HMOs.

- **CED recommends that employers increase consumer choice by offering employees a wide range of health plans and delivery systems. To achieve the benefits of competing approaches, it is essential that employer contributions to the cost of all plans be the same fixed-dollar amount rather than the full cost of all plans or a constant proportion of all premiums.**

Small firms may have more difficulty in offering a full range of choice than large companies. This problem could be overcome if groups of small employers combine their resources through multiemployer insurance plans.

The concept of a wider choice among health plans has been expanded to include choosing the mix of health and nonhealth benefits such as pensions. These *cafeteria plans* were permitted by amendments to the Internal Revenue Code in 1978. In 1982, the introduction of the *flexible spending account* carried the concept a step further by permitting employees to place pretax dollars into accounts from which medical and other expenses, such as child care and legal services, could be paid. Unspent balances in these accounts at the end of the year could be taken in cash. But in 1984, this cash-out feature was suspended by Internal Revenue Service regulations. There clearly should be a balance between the desirability of greater options for employees to select a fringe benefit package that meets their needs and unnecessarily generous opportunities to shelter income not used for actual medical expenses.

We believe that the concept underlying the cafeteria plan should be retained, at least to the extent that it permits employees to exercise greater choice of health insurance coverage. However, employers and their insurance carriers must design options so that the concept of spreading risk among a diverse group of employees is not eroded by adverse selection.

INCENTIVES TO CONSTRAIN COSTS

- **We believe that employer-based health plans should require employees to pay at least part of the cost when the service is used. This does not mean that all the options offered have to include cost sharing. In a market-based system, it is appropriate to offer the choice of a plan with no cost sharing; but in this case, the plan should carry an additional premium paid by the employee.**

It is important that consumers have a choice among plans, one or more of which have some significant cost-sharing features, and that they assume financial responsibility for making costlier choices. In other words, if an employee would like a plan with little or no cost sharing and is *willing to contribute to the higher premium that would be associated with such a plan,* there is good reason to allow that individual this option. The problem with traditional arrangements for purchasing group health insurance through the workplace is that either plans with significant cost sharing were not offered, or they were offered in a way that clearly made them unattractive to employees. With the employer paying most or all of the extra premium amount for the alternative plan with less cost sharing, there was no incentive for employees to select plans with cost-sharing features. Thus, the essence of the market approach is to establish the principle that if you want a little extra, you pay a little extra. *Extra* in this context might mean either a policy with no cost sharing or a policy with the same degree of cost sharing as the other plans offered but some extra coverage for services such as eyeglasses and dental care.

In response to rising health care costs, Air Products and Chemicals, Inc., substituted coverage with deductibles at the point when services are used for first-dollar coverage and at the same time introduced more complete health coverage for very large medical bills (see page 45). This combined better cost discipline for routine outlays with better protection against unusually large expenses. The Air Products plan also illustrates the benefits of tailoring optional delivery systems to each plant in a multiplant company.

It is important to distinguish between cost sharing for extra coverage, (see "Cost-Sharing Techniques at Household International," page 46) and cost sharing at point of service use. While it is desirable to bring the cost of care to the attention of the patient so that he or she is not indifferent to the gap between high and low price tags, it is also important to shield lower-income people from a cost-sharing burden that they could not afford. Unaffordable cost sharing will lead patients to forgo needed care, which is clearly undesirable. Thus, it is important to scale the degree of cost sharing to the resources of the beneficiary. Indeed, some companies, such as Xerox Corporation, have developed cost-sharing requirements that vary with employee salary levels.

- **Given the influential role employers exercise in shaping the demand for health care services and improving the information available to the consumers of the services, CED recommends that employers develop utilization review mechanisms as an integral part of their health plans.**

A common employer response to rising health care costs is to participate in the management of the delivery of care to employees. Some employers attempt to minimize unnecessary use of services through utilization reviews (see "Health Care Innovations at General Motors Corporation," page 48). Generally speaking, these innovations are developing within the context of traditional financing arrangements. Frequently, these measures attempt to limit utilization within the fee-for-service system in ways that leave the basic method of payment intact.

In recent years, the most common forms of utilization control have been *preadmission certification* for hospitalization, *second-opinion programs* for surgery, and *concurrent stay review* that limits the length of stay in

A REDESIGNED HEALTH PLAN AT AIR PRODUCTS AND CHEMICALS

Medical cost increases at a compound annual rate of 17 percent for the 1979-1984 period at Air Products and Chemicals, Inc., prompted the introduction of a redesigned medical plan in 1985. The company's cost-management strategy involved (1) reexamination of the role played by its insurance carriers; (2) involvement of local, state, and national coalitions that play a role in the development of public policy on health care costs and delivery; and (3) corporate introduction and sponsorship of wellness, fitness, and safety programs for employees and their families.

In the redesigned plan, the notion of a reasonable level of up-front deductibles coupled with cost sharing for all expenses in excess of the deductibles (up to a moderate limit on out-of-pocket outlays, sometimes referred to as a *stop-loss provision*) was substituted for first-dollar coverage. A new Medical Advisory Program (MAP) for hospital precertification and an advisory and referral service were introduced. MAP coordinates the delivery of some new services under the plan, such as hospice care, alcohol and drug abuse treatment, home health care, and fully paid second surgical opinions. It also steers employees toward quality services. Air Products offers an HMO option in locations where this is a viable alternative, and to date between 30 percent and 50 percent of the eligible employees have enrolled.

The examination of insurance carriers by Air Products had three results: (1) It was decided that the company was best served by self-insuring its medical costs. (2) It was determined that more attention was needed to the manner in which carriers paid claims. (3) It was found that the carriers' data claims systems were rudimentary. Changes are being made to ensure that appropriate utilization data will be available on a timely basis.

Air Products has made a major commitment to promoting healthy and safe lifestyles for its employees and their families. Programs such as smoking cessation, high blood pressure screening and management, aerobic exercise, and driver safety have been available for the past several years. Recently, the company has completed construction of a fitness center at headquarters.

The best indicator of the success of innovations at Air Products is the impact on the year's health care costs. In 1985, health care costs grew at the rate of overall inflation. Beyond this, the company believes those employees who use MAP are becoming better consumers of health care and that cost sharing can induce employees to consider changes in the delivery of health care.

46

an institution that will be reimbursed. These approaches are sometimes combined with financial incentives in the form of reduced cost sharing to encourage the performance of certain medical procedures on an outpatient basis.

A 1983 survey of 250 employee benefits officers in Fortune 500 companies conducted by Louis Harris and Associates for the Equitable Life

---

COST-SHARING TECHNIQUES AT HOUSEHOLD INTERNATIONAL

At Household International, a multi-industry corporation (transportation, finance, and manufacturing), senior management has for the past two or three years expressed a strong desire to provide adequate health care benefits for employees without letting the cost of those benefits become a major runaway factor. The company undertook a study of the problem and determined that benefits should be restructured so that the employee population could assist the company in controlling the overall health care bill. The restructured program was implemented at Household International and its financial services subsidiaries on January 1, 1985.

The key element of the new plan is the choice that employees must make among three medical plans. The high plan is similar to the prior program (i.e., first-dollar hospital and surgical coverage, low deductibles) but with a large increase in the required level of the employee's contribution. At the other extreme, the low plan, with sharply higher deductibles and coinsurance, is available for a nominal contribution. The company also offers a middle option in terms of deductibles and level of contribution. All three plans include specific cost-containment elements such as mandatory second surgical opinions, coverage for hospice and certain home health care services as alternatives to hospital care, features to encourage the use of outpatient services, and restrictions on nonemergency weekend hospital admissions. All employee contributions to each plan are made with pretax dollars.

Household's objective was to give employees a financial incentive (missing in the past) to buy only the coverage really needed and to utilize the most cost-effective treatments appropriate to the problem being treated.

Household has been pleased to date with its new plan. Approximately 32 percent of employees elected a lower level of medical coverage in 1985 than they had under the prior plan. These employees now have an incentive to be more cost-conscious in their utilization of medical services, which will yield cost savings without lowering the quality of care received. Employees can also determine for themselves how much medical insurance they should purchase. The firm has had very positive comments from employees on this point.

Assurance Society found that 63 percent of the companies responding encouraged ambulatory settings for medical tests and minor surgery, 52 percent required second opinions for some surgery, 42 percent had third-party payers conduct utilization reviews, and 24 percent required insurance company approval of payment for specific expenses and lengths of stay prior to nonemergency hospitalization.[5]

Another 1983 survey, by A. S. Hansen Company, looked at small and medium-sized firms as well as larger companies.[6] It found that 20 percent of the companies either required or encouraged second opinions for surgery (a lower figure than the proportion of larger companies cited in the Harris survey), and that 80 percent of the companies had some type of voluntary second-opinion program. (Many experts believe that voluntary second-opinion programs have little or no payoff but that mandatory programs are cost-effective.) The Hansen survey also found that half of the companies had utilization review procedures as a condition for claims payment, and that a quarter of them restricted payment for unnecessary hospital admissions or excessive lengths of stay.

Until recently, the purchasers of care always seemed to give the providers the benefit of the doubt when it came to the use of the health care system at the margin. But as utilization is cut back, there is some danger of going too far. Some restrictions on utilization intended only to eliminate wasteful services could turn out to eliminate needed care. It is possible to classify high-cost care of questionable or marginal value as excessive or unnecessary. But in some cases, high-cost care can produce benefits significantly greater than the cost. The position one takes on such an issue may depend on whether one's vantage point is that of the patient, the insurance subscriber, the company, the government, or society as a whole. Most of the cost-benefit studies of second opinions on surgery have looked mainly at the benefits when the second opinion reverses an initial recommendation for surgery and have counted only the costs associated with paying for these second opinions, including time away from work. Largely neglected, indeed unmeasured, are the costs associated with a second opinion that is wrong but is followed. There are also cases where the initial opinion improperly recommends no surgery; in these cases, there would probably be no motivation to seek a second opinion. Mistakes involving a recommendation against surgery may take some time to be discovered (if they are discovered at all).

- **Although we support the trend toward utilization reviews, we recommend that health plans include a monitoring and evaluation program to ensure that employees are not denied access to services simply because the cost appears high.**

REDESIGNING BENEFIT PLANS FOR PROTECTION AGAINST CATASTROPHIC COSTS

Through major medical insurance, employer-based health plans now protect most workers and their families from incurring large economic losses when they require high-cost medical services. However, most Americans continue to be poorly protected for an illness that is chronic and

---

HEALTH CARE INNOVATIONS AT GENERAL MOTORS CORPORATION

Although General Motors and its major unions have differing views concerning the overall direction the health care delivery system should take to control costs, they both realize the need to work together to promote systematic change in the medical care system to control runaway health care costs. From this joint effort, a framework has emerged for a comprehensive first step toward effective cost containment measures.

In each national negotiation since 1970, the concept of employee involvement in controlling the cost of health care has been proposed to GM's major unions by GM management. The proposals included eliminating first dollar coverage of health care benefits by imposing copayments and deductibles at the time services are received, requiring employees to pay a portion of health care premiums, and implementing pilot cost containment programs. While the unions were willing to negotiate on the pilot programs, they remained emphatic in their rejection of proposals for employees sharing in the cost of basic health care coverages—maintaining that the cost would be a "cost transfer" to employees and that no reductions in total health care costs would occur.

Health care cost containment was first formalized in contract language as a joint GM and union objective in 1976. The initial approach called on the principal health care carriers to establish a system for hospital utilization review, to report on their activities, and to develop pilot programs, such as voluntary second opinion programs for surgery, hospital preadmission testing, and programs for independent monitoring of inpatient hospital care.

In the 1979 negotiations, the parties agreed to monitor more closely the hospital utilization review activities, develop a utilization review system for professional services and prescription drugs, and consider mandatory second opinion programs for certain surgeries.

By 1982, the economic condition of the auto industry and the continuing rise in health care costs forced both sides to seek common ground to reach agreement on health care cost containment. Among the pilot programs agreed to were the following: prior authorization and ambulatory surgery

requires long-term care or for acute care involving the use of innovations in medical procedures, such as organ transplants. The treatment of both types of illness now exposes even middle- and upper-income patients and their families to the elimination of a major portion of their assets.

Private markets have not dealt well with providing insurance protection for long-term care. Even though the government contributes heavily to the financing of long-term care for the poor, on average half of long-term

---

initiatives; maximum allowable cost generic drug substitution and mail order prescription drug programs; second surgical opinion programs; and prepaid (capitation) dental plans.

In an effort to promote both competition among providers and prudent purchasing decisions, GM and its major unions introduced the Informed Choice Plan (ICP) in April 1985. This program reflects the successes experienced through GM's numerous pilot programs and is a response to changing market conditions. ICP encourages employees to evaluate their needs with respect to various managed care options—such as the traditional option with predetermination and selective provider networks such as HMOs and PPOs.

Overall, 28 percent of GM's total health care contracts are participating in an HMO (17 percent) or PPO (11 percent), representing nearly 650,000 employees, retirees, and their dependents. More than 37 percent of GM's active employees have joined a managed care option. Initial evaluation indicates that the ICP is a success in terms of controlling runaway costs without compromising quality of care.

In addition, a 10 percent cost reduction target was introduced into carrier contracts in April 1985. Specific performance standards have been established for claims processing, payment accuracy, and statistical reporting such that carriers' reimbursement for administrative expenses is contingent upon the submission of accurate paid claims data.

GM also has developed two systems to track and verify data. The General Motors Claims System (GMCS), which all of GM's major carriers have implemented, verifies and tracks appropriate claims payment by the carriers. An internal management information system (MIS) was developed to monitor data aimed at isolating problems, tracking utilization and cost trends over time, and measuring program successes.

These efforts could not have occurred without the willingness and commitment of all parties to affect a joint campaign to contain health care costs. The Informed Choice Plan is an approach to cost containment that is compatible with maintaining an active interest in the ongoing quality of care.

care is paid for by users and their families. In 1977, the long-term care population was estimated at 6 million, most of whom required nonmedical rather than medical and unskilled rather than skilled care.[7]

Although about one-third of the long-term care population is under sixty-five years old, age is strongly associated with the need for such care. Less than 1 percent of the population under forty-five years requires this type of care, but the proportion rises to 32 percent of those over eighty-five.

Only about 25 percent of the elderly ever enter a nursing home, but for those who require long-term care, the cost can be catastrophic. Public health programs give only limited assistance. Medicare explicitly prohibits coverage of custodial care, and those who are eligible for skilled nursing home care usually exhaust their benefits before leaving the nursing home. Benefits for financing long-term care are available under Medicaid, but only if all other sources of personal income and wealth have been used. For the nonpoor, assistance for nursing homes is potentially available, but they must first exhaust their personal finances. All levels of government are concerned that more liberal standards of eligibility for public programs for long-term care will lead to an explosion in the use of custodial care outside of the nursing home. In a period of large federal budget deficits and the potential future insolvency of the Medicare program, there is little that the public sector can do on its own to increase its contribution to financing the health care needs of the current generation of the long-term care population.

- **CED recommends that the private and public sectors seek innovations in financing that will assist those requiring long-term care.**

Over the next two decades, individuals and their families will bear the heaviest burden of financing long-term care, but innovations in private-sector financing and public policy could provide some assistance. In order to respond to the problem of access to long-term care for the current generation of elderly, both private-sector actions and public policy should encourage innovations that attempt to link currently available public funds within a *managed-care institutional arrangement*. One of the most serious impediments to financing long-term care is the phenomenon of moral hazard: the likelihood that insurance coverage for health care service will result in a greater use of health care than if the insured were spending his or her own money. Under a managed-care arrangement, access to care can be controlled and limited to medical need. The current experiments with social HMOs, which cover the full range of ambulatory, acute inpatient, rehabilitative, nursing home, home health, and personal care under a prospectively determined fixed budget, appear promising. For low-income people ineligible for Medicaid, the social HMO receives a monthly premium from Medicare and an additional premium from the enrollees.

There are, of course, other institutional arrangements such as continuing care retirement communities, which are attempting to provide a full range of health services and long-term care to the elderly. All these arrangements have the advantage of responding to the current problem. They also provide a larger risk pool, which in the long run should make it more feasible for insurance companies to market long-term care insurance.

Another potential source of funding for long-term care is the vast equity that older homeowners have accumulated through totally or substantially paid-off mortgages. The total value of this equity has been estimated at $700 billion. Elderly homeowners could receive a flow of income through home equity conversion arrangements under which they pledge a portion of the value of their house in return for *reverse mortgage payments*. Numerous barriers to participation in this arrangement are faced by both the elderly and financial institutions, but given the magnitude of this source of untapped wealth, the concept deserves careful study.

The growing proportion of elderly in the population will unquestionably lead to an increased demand for public programs for financing long-term care for the nonpoor elderly. Among the elderly, those seventy-five and older have the greatest need for long-term care. In 1980, 39 percent of the elderly were older than seventy-four years; by 2000, this proportion will rise to 49 percent. Any attempt to expand public programs to meet the expected increased demand will require either higher Social Security taxes for the working population or a reallocation of government health care expenditures toward those requiring long-term care and away from other services.

Although CED would not rule out more effective use of public expenditures to assist in the financing of long-term care for a greater proportion of the elderly, we believe that an additional tax on the working population for this purpose would be inequitable and detrimental to the future growth of the economy.

Another option for meeting the expenses associated with long-term care is *individual medical accounts* (IMAs), which are similar to individual retirement accounts (IRAs). This option, which has been proposed by the Department of Health and Human Services, would encourage people to save for these expenses during their working years. As with IRAs, the interest earned on the savings would not be taxed as it accumulates. IMAs could help fund long-term care without incurring any tax liability at the time of withdrawal. Any unused balance in the account would be transferred to an individual's estate.

Such approaches should be seriously considered. However, CED has consistently taken the position that in the current budget environment, it is essential to identify clearly how such proposals would be financed.

- **CED believes that the most appropriate solution to the problem is likely to come from freestanding long-term care insurance and/or the integration of such insurance within employee benefit packages.**

The threat of an explosion of the demand for long-term care services by the beginning of the next century is a serious problem, but it also presents the private sector with the opportunity to do something now. If employers can make employees aware of the fact that they are at risk of exposure to catastrophic long-term care costs which government programs will not cover, they will, we believe, prompt individuals to take action to protect themselves. If the private sector can develop benefit policies that ensure employees the opportunity to purchase long-term care insurance starting some fifteen to twenty years before retirement, it is likely that the premium cost will be affordable for most people.

Employers can help stimulate the growth of insurance for this type of care. Indeed, a number of insurance carriers have started to offer coverage for care for as long as five years, and some have offered such policies through private institutions that provide a full range of managed care for the elderly.

CED welcomes these initiatives by the insurance industry but believes that the private sector must take the initiative in redesigning benefit plans to ensure that a long-term care insurance component is available to employees before they are close to retirement. Where it is available today, long-term care insurance generally only fills in some of the cost-sharing requirements under Medicare. Moreover, it is generally marketed to *older individuals*, rather than to *employee groups,* and the typical policy contains a number of restrictions such as a requirement of a prior hospitalization. Under these conditions, *adverse risk selection* is likely to occur, with only older employees or retirees with a high probability of requiring long-term custodial care electing coverage.

An alternative would be to redesign employee benefit policies, in conjunction with collective bargaining practices where appropriate. Some existing benefit packages could be traded for long-term care protection. If employee groups showed this kind of interest, insurance carriers might have a greater incentive to market this type of insurance.

- **CED recommends that two components of current health care plans might be traded for the introduction of long-term care coverage: employer-paid group life insurance and health benefits for retirees.**

REDUCTION OF EMPLOYER-PAID GROUP LIFE INSURANCE
Employee needs for group life insurance vary with age. From the employee's perspective, for example, the need for life insurance may diminish with age while the demand for insurance against the catastrophic

cost of long-term illness is likely to increase. In order to avoid a simple add-on to the already high cost of fringe benefits, it may make more sense for employers to offer to gradually phase down their contribution to employee life insurance after employees reach a specific age and transfer part of the premium saving to long-term care insurance.

One cautionary note is necessary here: if employers begin to phase down life insurance coverage for workers at too young an age in order to get out in front of the adverse selection problem for long-term care, they might reduce life insurance coverage when workers still need it. With many people having children later in life, the need for life insurance protection may remain strong for a longer period than in the past. Thus, we need to balance the various needs of workers in their forties, fifties, and sixties to achieve a proper degree of risk reduction.

REVISING AND RESTRUCTURING BENEFITS FOR RETIREES

Many employer plans now provide substantial health insurance benefits for retired employees. In some circumstances it may be desirable to scale down current benefits for retirees where this can be legally done in return for long-term care protection.

In addition, employers can experiment with better integration of acute and long-term care benefits. Some companies are now considering pooling arrangements in which the money Medicare would pay on behalf of their retirees is merged with company retirement benefits designed to fill in some of the gaps left by Medicare. Generally speaking, both Medicare and private employer coverage do not include long-term care. Through introducing better cost management and utilization review into the acute care coverage, however, a manager of a pooled fund might be able to extend a greater measure of long-term care coverage. Government-sponsored social HMO experiments are testing this concept.

Some employers may wish to incorporate long-term care protection into a cafeteria approach, with the available menu of types of coverage varying with age. For example, younger persons might be eligible for some dental coverage that would be phased out as long-term care coverage is introduced.

The technical difficulties of overcoming the basic problems of moral hazard and adverse selection associated with long-term care insurance preclude any simple solution. Nevertheless, the private sector has a responsibility to act now. Moreover, in a pluralistic health care strategy, government also has a responsibility to seek innovations in the financing and provision of long-term care.

Much can be done to alter the priorties under Medicare without mounting a major increase in total expenditures. A greater measure of protection for long-term care could be built into Medicare and paid for by increased beneficiary contributions. Such contributions could take the form of either more complete taxation of Medicare benefits or higher Medicare premiums adjusted for income.

- **CED recommends that consideration be given to redesigning the current Medicare program to finance a greater measure of protection for long-term care in a managed care environment.**

FINANCING ACCESS TO HIGH-COST MEDICAL INNOVATIONS

The private sector has performed extremely well in providing insurance against most catastrophic costs associated with acute illness. Nevertheless, under the pressure of rising costs, some employer-based plans have limits. For some with serious illnesses, there is a gap in coverage, especially when the treatment may be considered experimental. Advances in medical science (such as organ transplants) have provided major potential health benefits but are frequently not covered by insurance plans.

Decisions on the type of procedures covered under Medicare also have important implications for the efficient distribution of public funds to achieve the maximum health benefits for society. The current proposal to make heart transplants available under Medicare raises serious economic and social issues. Public expenditure on health care is an investment. Is the social return from an investment in high-cost organ transplant maximized by investing public funds to provide benefits to those eligible for Medicare? Is it equitable for others requiring similar medical treatment to be denied access simply because they are not part of that group?

As new procedures and treatments prove relatively successful, they are usually added as reimbursable under public and private plans. Although this incremental response to potentially high-cost innovations has proven reasonably successful, more significant changes may be needed.

- **CED recommends that private plans consider including both major medical coverage and one or more additional riders to the basic policy permitting the purchase of additional insurance. The premium for this additional insurance rider could include a significant degree of cost sharing, with the amount paid by the employee based on salary.**

Riders can be applied to a wide range of services, including some high-cost services with a low probability of occurrence, such as organ transplants, long-term care for the frail elderly, and long-term care for severe psychiatric disorders. Or a rider might cover routine and relatively inexpensive services not included in the basic policy, such as dental services and eyeglasses. Cost sharing in the purchase of coverage for additional services would be entirely consistent with a market-driven system of health care. It would also be preferable to the inevitable tendency for government, usually at the state level, to mandate the specific services to be included in an employee health care package.

PRIVATE-SECTOR RESPONSIBILITY FOR THE MEDICALLY INDIGENT

More extensive reliance on market incentives in health care will make the problem of providing a reasonable minimum level of access to health care for everyone much more visible. The private sector currently contributes to this goal by financing a substantial part of the health costs of senior citizens through employer and employee payroll taxes earmarked to the Medicare program. Many employers also provide retiree health benefits that cover a portion of the elderly's health care cost that Medicare does not cover. In the past employees and employers also subsidized indigent care through additional charges on hospital and doctor bills over and above the cost of services actually consumed.

As government attempts to contain cost increases in the Medicare and Medicaid programs, and as employers become more cost-conscious buyers in health care markets, the complex system of subsidies for indigent care will be eroded. Consequently, there will be increased pressure for the government to develop a more explicit approach to financing indigent care. Under market-driven policies, however, the private sector has an opportunity to ease the pressure by reducing the size of the indigent care population.

Some people who resort to indigent care have health insurance, but the combination of this insurance and their savings does not cover their medical bills. But most of the medically indigent are uninsured or have only limited insurance protection. About three-fourths of the uninsured are in families with an employed head of the household. Many of these workers are employed by small firms that do not offer group health insurance. The extremely high cost of purchasing health insurance at nongroup rates precludes these workers from taking care of their families on their own. This is not a realistic option for reducing the proportion of uninsured employees.

The size of the medically indigent population would be reduced significantly if private-sector business groups, such as local chambers of commerce and health care coalitions, working with insurance companies, could offer group health insurance to small employers and individuals. One vehicle for achieving this goal is the multiemployer trust. Another approach involves state-wide risk pools. Sponsors of these types of group plans would, of course, need to establish rules that prevent adverse selection through individual employees entering and leaving the plan according to their own or their dependents' medical condition.

- **As part of the solution to the problem of financing indigent care, CED urges private-sector groups to take this type of initiative in extending insurance coverage to employees whose employer does not now offer group health insurance.**

In addition to pooling risks and resources, employers can help in several other ways. For example, in negotiations with hospitals and other medical care providers, they can recognize the uncompensated cost of indigent care as a legitimate part of provider overhead. Although no one employer could reasonably be asked to underwrite such uncompensated cost, sharing a portion of this cost among a large number of bill payers could address the problem of revenue shortfalls without creating an undue burden.

Suppose that an insurer or a self-insured employer is bargaining with a hospital over the size of the discount that will be allowed from normal hospital charges. An employer with a large number of workers in that particular geographic area or an insurer with a large pool of subscribers can exercise a great deal of leverage to extract a significant discount. Increasingly, such market strength translates into saying, "If you want the right to serve our 10,000 employees, you will have to get your price down closer to the actual cost of serving them." Such bargaining often boils down to what items of overhead this buyer will agree to fund on a pro rata basis.

At this juncture, an employer could agree to shave a percentage point off the discount that could otherwise be extracted from the provider. Thus, a discount of 12 percent might be reduced to 11 percent, so that the employer pays 1 percentage point more than it might otherwise find necessary to pay.

This type of strategy is not meant to be a long-term solution to the indigent care problem. As explained in Chapter 6, such a solution involves a fundamental overhaul of our public assistance system and entails important roles for government and the private sector. The point here is to encourage employers and providers to take interim steps that alleviate the hardship associated with indigent care until a long-term solution is found.

Business leaders should recognize that they often pay a portion of the cost of uncompensated health care *anyway*. As payers of property taxes, for example, they incur a portion of the cost of supporting a local public hospital that must serve a rising number of nonpaying patients. And as income taxpayers (state and federal), they may pay higher taxes to finance government payments to improve Medicaid benefits.

We favor public-sector reforms that would end some of the gross inequities in current indigent care programs. It is unrealistic, however, to expect government to pay for the full health care costs of every low-income person. If it did, some employers of low-wage workers who now provide health insurance might eliminate their coverage and shift this cost onto government. What is needed is a blended strategy that involves some measure of Medicaid reform or subsidized risk pools at the state level and a private-sector contribution. If the private system is strengthened as the public coverage system is incrementally expanded, this important problem could be solved without a major shift toward a government-imposed solution.

Employers can also contribute to the solution through their involvement with local hospitals. Many business leaders serve as hospital trustees and thus can bring management expertise to the hospital and build a bridge between the buyer and seller sides of the hospital market.

PROVIDER RESPONSES TO MARKET INCENTIVES

As the buyers of health care tighten up and restructure the payment system, suppliers of health care are responding accordingly. The organization and delivery of health care are changing in ways designed to build a greater measure of cost consciousness into the system.

CHANGES IN THE DELIVERY SYSTEM

There has been a sharp growth in group practices of physicians. In 1970, only 16.4 percent of physicians were in group practices; as of November 1983, an estimated 38.5 percent of nonfederal, office-based physicians in the United States were practicing in groups of three or more. [8] These practices, through close-knit peer review and established referral patterns, can help to improve the efficiency of the health care system.

Although HMOs, one form of group practice, still constituted only 7 percent of total enrollment in health plans in 1984, they have grown rapidly in recent years. Nationwide, about forty new HMOs were formed between mid-1983 and mid-1984, and thirty-four more were added during the last six months of 1984. [9] HMOs are now starting to sign up Medicare enrollees in significant numbers after years of negligible enrollment of senior citizens; the increase between June 1983 and June 1984 was 36 percent. [10] This can be expected to accelerate further under Medicare's new policy governing contracting with HMOs and other competitive medical plans.

There has also been a tremendous increase in outpatient surgery. Although much of this surgery occurs in physicians' offices or hospital outpatient departments, there are now about 250 freestanding surgery centers in the United States, about double the number that existed in 1980. Several studies suggest that these centers perform high-volume surgical procedures at a lower cost than hospitals do on an inpatient basis.[11] Thus, their existence may pressure competitors to bring down their charges.

The growth in outpatient surgery has been facilitated by dramatic technological change. Many insurance plans encourage outpatient procedures. Some benefit packages now cover only 80 percent of inpatient charges for procedures that could be done on an outpatient basis but will cover 100 percent of the outpatient charges which are generally lower.

GREATER SPECIALIZATION AND REGIONALIZATION OF SERVICES

The spread of prospective payment systems and a variety of utilization review measures will put pressure on the providers of care, particularly hospitals, to specialize in services for which they can keep costs below reimbursable amounts, and to move out of services for which they cannot bring costs in line with payments. For example, hospitals may find that their cardiologists are keeping their budgets within Medicare's amounts but that, despite their best efforts at management reform, their orthopedic surgeons are exceeding reimbursements from Medicare, Blue Cross, and other insurers. It is reasonable to expect that over time this hospital will begin to specialize in cardiac surgery and move away from orthopedic surgery.

More specialization of services, based on both quality and cost, will lead to a greater regionalization of health services. Certain hospitals will be the centers for certain services for larger regions. Innovations in the way patients gain access to the system, ranging from helicopter transport to the development of satellite centers with feeder and referral networks of specialized facilities, will improve health service delivery.

These trends will be reinforced by the growing interest in measuring the quality of care. The U.S. Department of Health and Human Services issued new regulations in 1985 that will give the public access to information on the quality of patient care in hospitals. Mortality rates for various procedures will be made available to the public, and both patients and those who help pay their bills can examine this comparative information. Working through professional review organizations, the government will also provide information on the frequency with which a given procedure is performed, the average length of hospital stay, postoperative infection rates, and the cost of various procedures.

Of course, there will be a need to adjust such information for the special circumstances of various hospitals just as DRG rates must be adjusted for hospitals that have different case mixes. For example, a particular hospital may have a higher mortality rate because it admits relatively sicker patients with more complications. There is a need for caution in organizing and "cleaning" the data so that hospitals do not have a built-in incentive to avoid admitting the more serious or complicated cases.

As information on the quality of patient care filters through the community, patients will want to use the hospitals with the best performance records. This will lead to higher occupancy rates in the high-quality hospitals and lower rates in hospitals with less favorable records. In fact, the very concept of a hospital may change, and the full-line community hospital that offers some of everything may gradually disappear.

All this readjustment, of course, will not occur without opposition or delays. Communities will sometimes recoil at the prospect of closing certain wings of a hospital or closing the hospital altogether despite the hospital's comparative disadvantage in the provision of particular services. Some areas may prefer less than optimal but readily available services to a shortage that requires patients to travel a substantial distance to obtain care.

Moreover, there are certain barriers to the realignment of service provision along the lines of economic efficiency and quality. For example, the lack of hospital staffing privileges at the higher-performing hospital may preclude some physicians from admitting their patients there. Such barriers may be overcome as either the doctors obtain admitting privileges or patients switch to doctors that already enjoy this status.

The growing ratio of physicians to the population should facilitate greater specialization in the delivery system and make physicians more open to new organizational forms. As doctors fight to obtain a full patient load, they will align themselves more with specific hospitals and become a part of more fully integrated health care systems.

CED believes that efforts to utilize market-oriented incentives in order to hold down health care costs are beneficial and should be further strengthened and developed. However, as competitive pressures erode inefficient cross-subsidies and bring costs down certain problems may occur. These include an underemphasis on technological development and product innovation and an inadequate system of protection for those who lack the resources (or the good health) to participate effectively in a market system. Basic research may be underfunded because firms cannot capture the returns from such investments. Moreover, competitive forces may cause providers to avoid patients who cannot pay for services because these unreimbursed costs cannot readily be passed along to paying customers. These concerns are valid, but we believe that they should not be used to delay or thwart the reliance on market forces. Specific policies must be devised to assure that these needs are addressed even as competition and deregulation in health care markets continue to be stressed.

Chapter 5

Innovation in Medical Devices, Procedures, and Pharmaceuticals

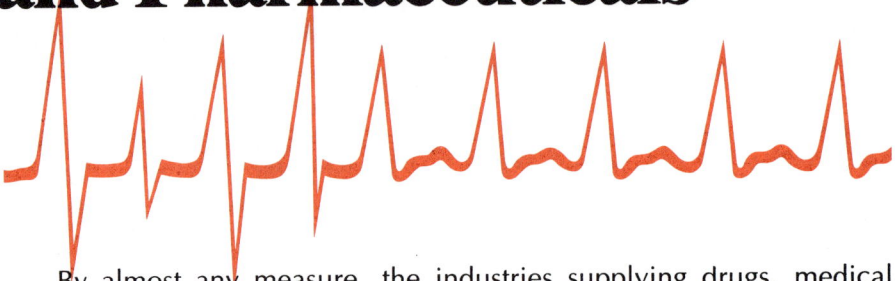

By almost any measure, the industries supplying drugs, medical devices, and professional medical knowledge and skill have traditionally been highly innovative. As with other industries, the stimulus for innovations comes from the economic return generated by the increased productivity the innovation produces. If a new drug, device, or procedure can reduce the cost of an existing treatment or produce a more effective treatment, there is an incentive for suppliers to innovate if there is an opportunity to earn sufficient profit.

INNOVATION IN A REGULATED MARKET[1]

Government intervention strongly influences the health care market. Therefore, decisions on how and for what services the government reimburses providers inevitably shape how investments are made for the development of new drugs, devices, and procedures. The type of reimbursement system associated with employer-based health plans also influences innovation.

The rapid growth of expenditures by business on health care services, stimulated by government incentives and direct government outlays, has significantly increased the demand for innovations. These innovations have improved treatment, and many have been cost-effective. At the same time, until recently the almost exclusive reliance on cost-based reimbursement by the government and third-party payers has also encouraged overutilization of some innovations when a less advanced and less costly technology would have been equally successful. In addition, the traditional reimbursement system has encouraged the use of innovations that make a positive contribution to health, but the cost of using the technology may outweigh any additional benefit to society — for example, when heroic efforts are made to preserve the life of a patient whose death is imminent.

Employers who sponsor health plans have a responsibility to act as a countervailing force to such overutilization. Working with insurance carriers, they should make cost-effectiveness reviews of medical innovations an integral part of utilization review. Similarly, by reviewing or conducting cost-effectiveness studies to determine whether specific devices and drugs will be approved for reimbursement under Medicare and Medicaid, the government can minimize unnecessary use.

At the same time, cost-effectiveness studies should recognize the fact that the short-run cost of any innovation is an inappropriate indicator of unnecessary utilization. While the innovation is experimental or not yet widely available, its cost per patient use is likely to be high. Consequently, evaluations should consider costs in the context of the potential long-term net benefits.

Since the beginning of this century, the supply of health care innovations, especially drugs, has been regulated by the government. It is widely accepted that some form of regulation is necessary to protect public health. Drugs, devices, and advances in procedures should be acceptably safe and effective; they should produce the diagnostic and therapeutic effects claimed. Safety and effectiveness should be evaluated on the basis of well-controlled experiments judged by qualified experts.

Studies of the costs and benefits of many important new drugs and technologies have demonstrated that medical innovations can make important contributions to the reduction of health care costs and the eradication or control of infections and communicable diseases. The interrelationship between the development of drugs and devices has combined with improved professional skills to produce remarkable advances in medical practice.

THE SLOWDOWN IN INNOVATIONS

Since the beginning of the 1970s, regulatory policies significantly slowed pharmaceutical innovation. More recently, regulatory policies have unnecessarily hampered the introduction of new devices. New drugs and medical technologies have produced substantial benefits, but as overall costs have escalated, the contribution of innovations in the drug industry to improved efficiency of health care appears to have declined.

Drugs and medical sundries now account for less than 7 percent of total health care system costs, compared with 12 to 13 percent in 1965. During the 1970s, drug prices increased at a substantially lower rate than the Consumer Price Index for medical commodities and the overall rate of inflation. This lower rate is due largely to the strong productivity in the pharmaceutical preparation and drugstore industries during the 1965-1974 period,[2] when productivity grew at an average annual rate of about 5 percent for pharmaceuticals and about 6 percent annually in the drugstore industry. But between 1974 and 1981, average productivity growth in pharmaceuticals dropped to 2 percent, and drugstore productivity growth declined to less than 2 percent.

Without the high productivity in drugs and medical sundries during the early 1970s, the escalation of health care costs would have been greater. Although productivity growth is still higher in the drug and medical sundries sector than in the rest of manufacturing, the sharp decline by the mid-1970s is cause for considerable concern.

U.S. preeminence in pharmaceutical innovation has been declining. The average number of new chemical entities is a good indicator of the technological ability to submit new drugs for FDA approval. In a study of the average annual number of new chemical entities tested in humans by thirty-nine U.S. pharmaceutical firms, it was found that from 1977 to 1979 only twenty-six such entities were tested, half the average annual rate during the previous decade.[3] As Figure 1 demonstrates, the development of new drugs in foreign countries has increased sharply since 1963; by 1980, the average annual rate of foreign-tested new chemical entities had converged with the U.S. rate.

STIMULATING INNOVATIONS

The influence of government policy on the rate of innovation depends on the type of medical product or procedure and on the phase of the innovation process most affected by government policy.

PHASES OF THE INNOVATION PROCESS

The first phase, *basic research*, encompasses studies of the fundamental elements and processes of science. Typically, the motive of basic research is to acquire knowledge for its own sake, without serious regard for the possibilities of useful application. The second phase, *applied research*, strives to apply basic knowledge to the solution of a particular problem or need. Often the distinction between these two phases is more an intellectual exercise than a practical division; in reality, laboratory work flows from one experiment to another. Once an applicable idea is proven in a labora-

FIGURE I

New Drug Development by U.S. Firms

Number of self-originated NCEs entering clinical testing each year.

Percentage of those NCEs first studied in man abroad.

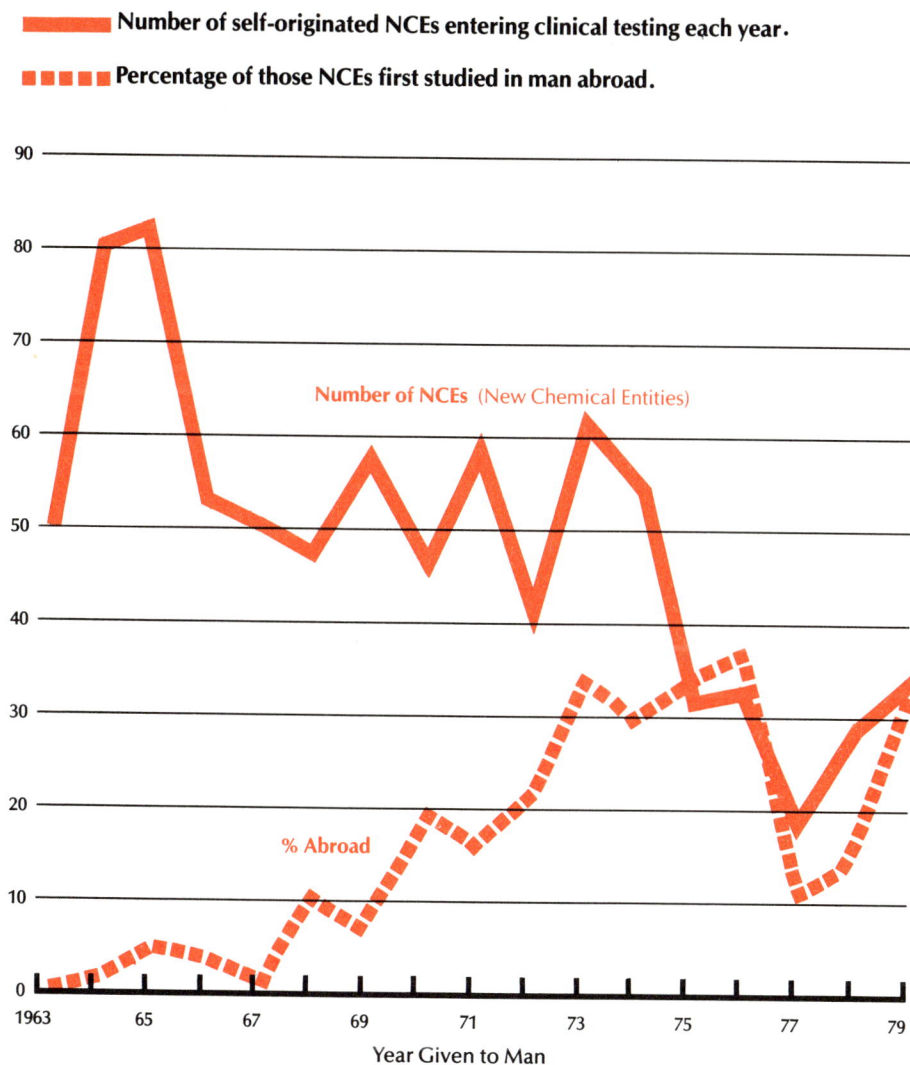

Number of NCEs (New Chemical Entities)

% Abroad

Year Given to Man

SOURCE: William M. Wardell, Maureen S. May, and A. Gene Trimble, "New Drug Development by United States Pharmaceutical Firms," *Clinical Pharmacology and Therapeutics* 32: 4 (October 1982), extracted from page 409.

tory setting, it must go through testing and refinement in the third stage, *development*.

Realizing the fruits of investment in these early stages of innovation requires a fourth phase in which applied knowledge is incorporated into a full-scale facility capable of producing the product or service. This *first-of-a-kind facility* must be supported by capital investment, access to raw materials, labor, energy, marketing facilities, and of course, consumer demand for the output.

The fifth phase is the *diffusion* of the innovation throughout the health care system. How fast this occurs will depend on such factors as market receptivity, competitive conditions, the age of existing capital stock, and the overall pace of demand for the innovation. The commercial application of the new technique, drug, or device is the stage of innovation that yields the greatest benefits to society. The market system provides the private sector with strong incentives to ensure that this phase is completed without government financial support.

The early phases of the process are especially important in the markets that supply products and services to the health care system. Improvements in medical procedures resulting from clinical practice in hospitals depend heavily on basic biomedical research. Even when applied clinical experiments produce successful new procedures, the result cannot usually be patented. Although patents, trademarks, and copyrights help ensure that the return from the investment accrues to the innovator, they do not guarantee that he or she will receive all the profits. Conversely, in a market-driven health care system, when ownership rights to innovation cannot be patented, there is little incentive for hospitals to engage in costly R & D.

In the early phases, innovations in medical devices also depend on R & D investment. But because the final result is typically a patentable product, innovators have some ability to capture and protect any return. Consequently, the private sector has an incentive to invest in applied R & D. For the medical device industry, the most important phases are the initial production of devices and the ability of management to market them as soon as possible. Premarketing approval and extensive adoption of a device produce economies of scale, which, in turn, permit the price to be lowered rapidly.

For pharmaceutical manufacturing, each phase in the process is important. Investment in R & D is especially large for the development of new drugs. These large up-front investments and the small proportion of new drugs actually marketed successfully make it necessary for developers to be able to count on the flow of revenue produced by successful drugs that remain on the market for an extended period of time. Although almost the entire cost of financing pharmaceutical innovations is made by the private sector, government policy can influence the rate at which innovation occurs.

GOVERNMENT'S ROLE IN ENCOURAGING ADVANCES IN MEDICAL PRACTICES

Of the $5.0 billion spent yearly on R & D by industry, most goes to applied research for the testing and development of new products. More than half of all funds invested in basic research ($12.8 billion in 1985) is supplied by the government. Investment in basic R & D in some segments of the drug industry, such as pharmaceuticals and chemicals, is necessary because it is likely to provide guidance on potential applications. Hospitals and medical research institutes are usually willing to use their resources to develop new procedures only if successful R & D results in a patentable product or medical procedure.

R & D in hospitals is heavily concentrated in about 120 teaching and research institutions. But developing new techniques depends heavily on clinical research using new devices, drugs, and surgical procedures, and this research increases the cost of treating patients. The average cost of treating a patient in a teaching hospital is more than twice the cost in a community hospital. It is estimated that about 27 percent (or $639 per patient) of this additional cost is attributable to the clinical research associated with the development of new medical procedures.[4]

Traditionally, these additional costs were offset directly by government grants to specific medical researchers and by the original DRG formula under Medicare. Some of these costs were indirectly covered by increasing the hospital charges for patients receiving routine care. The move toward a market-driven system has reduced this cross-subsidy because employer health plans are now directing patients requiring routine care toward low-cost providers. The government is also considering cutting the research component in the DRG Medicare formula.

The continued flow of new medical procedures is essential to future improvements in the quality of, and advances in, U.S. health care. There is no doubt that part of the lost funding for innovations in medical procedures can be made up through more efficient use of professional resources within research-based institutions. However, because such innovations are essentially public goods that are rapidly diffused throughout the health care system, the government should provide a more explicit funding mechanism to maintain developmental research. Joint ventures in the private sector could also be helpful in sharing the cost of advances in medical procedures.

CED believes that any new mechanism for supporting research at medical institutions should be consistent with the goal of competition among all hospitals engaged in clinical research.

- **The new mechanism could be funded through an earmarked budget within the National Institutes of Health. All hospitals, both teaching and nonteaching, would be eligible for research grants.**

Awards should be based on the importance of the problem and the potential innovation, as well as the professional quality of the research team. Compared with the traditional system of cross-subsidization, this type of bidding is likely to improve the efficiency of clinical research and stimulate the competition among a wider variety of institutions.

In much government-supported basic research, a complementary relationship exists between research and the education of medical scientists. The investment in highly skilled professionals, particularly physicians, is financed partly by the individuals themselves and partly through a complex array of public subsidies to educational institutions. The fact that tuition accounts for only about 6 percent of the income of medical schools indicates that the market for training physicians is dominated by government subsidies.[5] Because the introduction of market-driven public and private health care policies will erode the current subsidy to medical education, the current system of indirect subsides will have to be replaced with a more explicit system.

REMOVING UNNECESSARY REGULATORY BARRIERS TO INNOVATION IN MEDICAL DEVICES

Medical devices range from relatively simple items to extremely complex machines. Consequently, a large number of firms of widely varying sizes develop new technologies involving either inspired tinkering or significant investment in sophisticated research.

The device industry has only recently been subject to FDA regulation, and not all devices must meet the same regulatory requirements. Products considered clearly safe (Class I) are subject only to general controls on labeling, registration, and good manufacturing practices. Those with greater potential for harm (Class II) must also meet performance standards, and those with the greatest potential for harming users (Class III) require pre-marketing approval. Because many devices are designed for hospital use, changes in hospital reimbursements such as the DRGs may have a significant impact on their market. Most of the major new devices are not available for direct purchase by consumers. Some devices represent major capital expenditures, and are purchased by hospitals and clinics; their subsequent utilizations require a physician's referral. Other devices, such as hip replacements, are used or administered by physicians.

Regardless of how cost-effective they are, some medical devices may prolong life or reduce pain and suffering and improve the quality of life.

Others are clearly cost-effective, but as is typical with many complex medical technologies, their initial cost is high, and the benefits are not fully recognized at the time the technology is introduced. Frequently, experience with the product demonstrates additional uses, some of which are cost-effective and some of which are not.

There are two major inefficiencies in the current regulatory process for approving medical devices. The first involves duplication in technology assessment by the HCFA and the FDA.

Section 1862(a) of the Social Security Act requires that the HCFA cover "reasonable and necessary" medical and related services. Although "reasonable and necessary" has never been defined, it has come to mean "safe and effective."[6] As a result, the usual practice at the Office of Health Technology Assessment, when conducting technology assessments in support of its coverage recommendations, is to examine safety and effectiveness. Since the FDA also examines safety and effectiveness, there is some duplication in the activities of the government agencies.

Unnecessary delay is a second problem. In the past, the HCFA did not initiate a review of whether a new technology would be covered under Medicare until final FDA approval was granted. There now appears to be more willingness for HCFA to initiate an assessment prior to final approval. If assessment of new technologies by HCFA were initiated early in the regulatory cycle, the benefits of approved innovations in medical devices would become available to Medicare patients more rapidly.

CED recommends that as soon as a technology is submitted to the FDA for approval, HCFA should begin its assessment of whether the technology will be covered under Medicare reimbursement. Thus, if a technology is approved by the FDA, the product could be paid for by Medicare without further delay. A comparison of costs and benefits of using a new device is a legitimate criterion for HCFA to consider. But if HCFA delays initiating its assessment until after FDA approval, it discourages hospitals from using the innovation for Medicare patients. This can unnecessarily deny Medicare patients treatment with the devices for years. Our recommendation shifts responsibility for the safety of a new device to FDA and restricts HCFA's responsibility mainly to appropriateness of including it under the Medicare reimbursement system.

An alternative approach is to permit partial reimbursement of hospitals that use FDA-approved devices while HCFA continues its assessment. The partial payments would be made for two years or until the final funding decision is made. Although this concept would be an improvement over the present regulatory approval process, we believe the decision to include a new device within the current DRG reimbursement system should be made simultaneously with the FDA approval process.

STIMULATING PHARMACEUTICAL INNOVATION

For some pharmaceutical innovations, cost effectiveness is easy to demonstrate if the direct cost of the drug is less than the cost of alternative treatments and the new drug improves the quality of care for the patient. Cost-effectiveness studies of important and frequently used drugs demonstrate that pharmaceutical innovations can contribute to lower health care costs and improved quality of care.[7] In most instances the cost effectiveness is not known at the time the innovation is introduced. Initially, the product may be very expensive and the price could be expected to fall with increased experience or with modifications.

A new drug can be extremely cost effective compared to alternate forms of treatment, but at the same time increase the overall costs of health care. For example, the immunosuppressant, cyclosporine, has improved the outcome of organ transplantation significantly and several studies have shown it to be cost effective. The indirect effect of the drug, however, has been to dramatically increase the rate of organ transplantation — raising the overall cost of health care.

Whether organ transplantation itself is cost effective depends on a number of factors including the medical condition and age of the patient. For example, transplants for older people are less likely to pass a test of cost effectiveness than a similar procedure performed on a younger person. Determining the criteria to allocate these scarce medical resources will be extremely difficult. As a society, however, we must be prepared to make the difficult economic and moral decisions necessary to avoid using these innovations inefficiently.

Pharmaceutical innovations can make an important contribution to both the treatment of patients and cost constraint. For example, the development of the drug Tagamet has provided an effective treatment for ulcers that both saves money and often reduces the need for painful exploratory surgery. It is therefore of considerable concern that over the period from 1961 to 1980, the production of new drugs in the major drug-producing countries declined markedly. In 1961, 93 new drugs were developed, while by 1980, only 48 new drugs were introduced, a 48 percent decrease from 1961. This declining trend is especially evident in the United States. In 1961, U.S. research produced 31 new substances; in 1980, this number dwindled to 13.

Many studies, both by academics and by industry experts, have investigated the causes of this decline. A consistent finding is that regulation has had a significant negative effect.

Delay in the approval process has also reduced the value of drug patents. In 1984, the Drug Price Competition and Patent Term Restoration Act extended the patent life for pharmaceuticals. Application for a patent is made early in development, even before the initiation of the extensive clinical trials. Because of the time required for clinical trials, the expected patent life of a new drug by 1981 was only seven years after approval despite the fact that the patent life for all products is seventeen years. The 1984 act has a complicated procedure for determining the patent life extension. Generally, the extension is equal to the time spent in regulatory review for approval plus half the time spent in clinical testing. The extension of the patent term will probably encourage new drug development by ensuring a more reliable rate of return on R & D costs. At the same time, however, the act recognized the importance of generic drugs to constraining costs and made it easier to market a generic drug. One possible adverse side effect of a greater reliance on generic drugs is that it will reduce the rate of return for the development of new chemical entities, which are the basis for increasing the availability of new drugs.

The need for efficiency in the regulatory process and the requirements for that efficiency must be more widely recognized outside the regulatory agencies, the R & D community in the pharmaceutical industry, and the academic community. The benefits of efficiency are potentially great, and although recent FDA commissioners have acknowledged the importance of improving the approval process, current policies do little to help meet this goal.

The scientific and clinical studies necessary to establish the risks and benefits of pharmaceutical products are both complex and expensive.[8] In addition, they represent potential risks to persons who are study subjects. Perfect knowledge of all the risks and benefits of new drugs in clinical trials of manageable size and duration is simply unachievable. For example, a reaction to a drug occurring in 1 out of every 2,000 or 3,000 patients in a population could easily escape detection in clinical trials involving many thousands of patients. It is the function of continuing scientific scrutiny and clinical observation of marketed products to detect and establish the causes of such very low-probability events.

The strongest protection of societal and patient interest in the accuracy, completeness, and safety of pharmaceutical studies is provided by the ethics of the scientific community and the need of corporate sponsors of new products to protect their reputations. Tort law, product liability, professional liability, and informed-consent requirements of various institutions provide additional protection. Academic processes, including peer review before and after publication in scientific journals and during many studies, represent further safeguards. For all clinical testing of new pharmaceuticals, there are institutional review boards with oversight responsibilities for study design and patient safety. Finally, the FDA exercises oversight and judgment on study designs, the qualifications of researchers, review board operations, and the number and types of studies necessary to establish the safety and efficacy for a pharmaceutical. Once a sponsor of a new product or a new use for an older product believes that the product is safe and effective for its intended uses, a New Drug Application (NDA) or an amended NDA is submitted to the FDA.

It has been estimated that for every 10,000 compounds investigated by pharmaceutical firms for possible marketing, 10 pass the initial scientific scrutiny that leads to testing in human subjects. Of these 10, only 1 survives the clinical tests and reaches the market. The process typically requires six to eight years from the first test in a human subject to first shipment for sale.[9] The typical cost of each average new chemical entity reaching the market was estimated at $54 million in 1976,[10] and is believed to have risen to about $100 million in 1986.[11] If the various studies of the so-called drug lag[12] (the extra time required by the U.S. approval process compared with that of other national scientifically oriented approval processes) are correct, the extra year or so of "waiting to market" time would account for about $10 million of this cost. There is little evidence that this extra time has added to public safety.

The process inefficiency leading to the drug-lag cost is a serious threat to the institutions pursuing pharmaceutical R & D. A number of studies have indicated that the financial rate of return on such investment for the average new chemical entity is essentially about that available in bond markets, in spite of the high level of risk involved.[13] Of course, some new products achieve very favorable returns, and the hope for such results stimulates the process. However, **any reduction in the length of the regulatory process without loss of necessary safety or efficacy assurance will improve the flow of new products and their contribution to health care**.

Society pays for the drug lag when safe and effective new products are, in effect, withheld from the market. Reduced competition in pharmaceutical markets and the impediment to improvements in health care are significant societal costs. It is clearly in the public interest to minimize these costs in a way that is consistent with maintaining necessary safety and efficacy.

The inefficiency of the U.S. drug approval process may have kept some potentially harmful products off the market. But it has also imposed costs on some individuals by denying or delaying the availability of drugs which on balance promote public health and actually save lives.

Incremental administrative changes in the FDA approval process can improve efficiency. For example, improving the flow of information between research-based companies and the FDA and developing an electronic data transfer system to partially replace the current large-scale submission of written reports would make a small contribution to reducing the transaction costs. Improving the quantity and quality of the scientific personnel available to the FDA is also desirable. This could be achieved by involving qualified scientists from other government agencies (such as the National Institutes of Health) in the approval process. However, such management reforms will make only a marginal contribution to improved efficiency.

Significant improvements will result only from a clearer definition of the FDA's function in the drug approval process. The government has two distinct functions in protecting the public interest against the risk of unsafe drugs.

First, the drugs already on the market must be inspected to ensure that their quality meets the standards of chemical composition and stability over their shelf life and that the manufacturing process meets prescribed standards of purity and sterility. The FDA is clearly the appropriate organization to ensure that manufacturing and product quality are met and that the public is protected if existing drugs do not meet these technical standards.

Second, government's function is to protect the public interest by permitting the private sector to market new drugs that are safe. Whether drugs meet this standard is essentially a scientific decision to determine the drug's benefits to patients in relation to its potential risk. It is highly questionable whether the FDA has superior ability to perform this function. Indeed, in a political environment in which Congress is extremely reluctant to admit that there are always risks as well as benefits from new drugs, civil servants are likely to be biased against approval in order to avoid being blamed for approving a drug with any potential for adverse side effects. This is the fundamental reason for the regulatory delay in marketing new drugs that meet safety and efficacy standards.

- **In order to eliminate the bias against approval, CED recommends that independent scientific experts and the views of those who may benefit from access to a drug be given a role in the approval process.**

At present, the FDA makes some use of advisory committees of independent scientists to review the study results. As in the case of approval of new medical devices, we believe that the use of expert advisory panels should be mandatory. These panels of independent scientific experts would review all applications for new chemical entities, comment on the design of clinical trials, and participate in the final decision on approval for marketing. **The FDA should remain responsible for protecting public safety. But under certain conditions, it should be made more difficult for civil servants to disregard the views of the independent scientific experts on the review panels**. If, for example, a majority (perhaps three-fourths) of a panel felt that a drug was safe for marketing under specified conditions, the FDA would be required to present written justification of its scientific reasons for disagreeing with the majority members before denying approval. A similar justification would be required if the FDA approved a drug that a majority of the review panel felt had not met the tests of safety and effectiveness.

It is likely that the participation of outside experts, including representatives of the patients who may benefit from the new drug (as is permitted if the drug affects a small number of patients, as defined in the Orphan Drug Act) will eventually expedite the approval process.

- **An additional reform that can reduce regulatory delay is to require the FDA to specify in advance (during the design of the clinical trials) what outcome of the trials will be accepted as sufficient evidence for approvals.**

Any additional evidence should be required only if the FDA can demonstrate that new scientific knowledge justifies the need for more information on potential effects in order to ensure the public's safety. This change is consistent with what is required for approval of orphan drugs. It is likely to eliminate the tendency to delay approval decisions by requiring additional evidence that may be interesting and useful but is not central to determining the drug's safety and efficacy.

Deciding which drugs should be permitted to compete in pharmaceutical markets is essentially a scientific issue. Whether such products should be covered under Medicare or any private-sector health plan is an economic issue that the FDA should not confuse with the scientific decision to allow products to enter the market. If the public is to benefit from access to new drugs, our regulatory system should encourage market competition so long as the drugs meet the standards of safety and efficacy determined by the scientific community both within and outside the FDA.

Chapter 6

Adopting Market Incentives in Public-Sector Policies

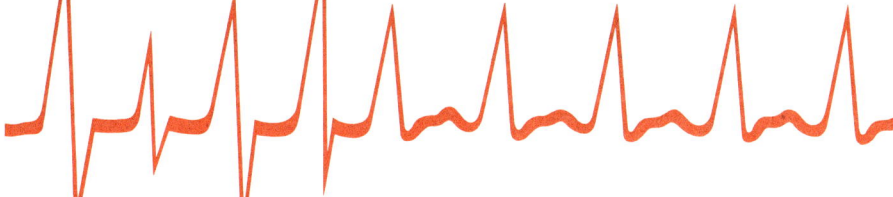

The central theme of the CED approach for reforming health care policies is the need to use market incentives in the implementation of both private-sector and public-sector policies. We believe that public as well as private health care systems can benefit from these incentives. In fact, when public policy incorporates market incentives, desired social objectives can be achieved with the least resources possible, freeing resources for alternative uses.

Building market incentives into public programs should be clearly distinguished from *privatizing* government programs. We are not advocating spinning off programs such as Medicare to the private sector or relying solely on private insurance for the elderly and low-income households. Rather, we believe that programs such as Medicare can be improved by building incentives for the cost-conscious use of resources. With greater use of incentives, the government's most important responsibility is to ensure an adequate financing mechanism for all those who are medically indigent.

As employers modify their health care plans so that employees become more cost-conscious, the cross-subsidies traditionally used to finance indigent care will be significantly reduced. Less heavily regulated health care markets will increase the need for a more effective safety net to catch those too poor or too ill to obtain adequate health insurance on their own.

In the past, most indigent care has been financed in two ways: through the Medicaid program, providing health insurance to a portion of the poor, and through a set of hidden subsidies under which low-income households ineligible for Medicaid were covered in a very indirect fashion. In effect, doctors and hospitals were expected to serve the poor regardless of their eligibility for Medicaid. The cost of charity care and bad debts was to be passed along to private-sector buyers through higher charges.

New developments in financing, especially the emphasis on cost containment and competition, are making it infeasible to load the costs of indigent care on top of the costs already carried by the private sector. It has now become necessary to transfer the medical costs of indigent sick people from sick people who are able to pay to society as a whole.

Armed with a new understanding of the health care marketplace and better information, employers are driving harder bargains with providers. An overbuilt hospital industry, facing substantial idle capacity and major restructuring, can no longer transfer the shortfall in public-sector payments for the indigent to the private sector.

The challenge is to devise new, direct, and efficient ways of subsidizing indigent care to take the place of the cross-subsidies that are rapidly being discarded. An additional challenge is to provide these subsidies while relying on market incentives rather than rigid government controls to achieve the best value possible for health care outlays.

Some will say the nation cannot afford such outlays. However, we believe that the choice is not really whether or not to pay for indigent care but, rather, whether to pay directly and openly or through more indirect, invisible mechanisms.

This is not to say that under the present system all health care needs are met. They are not, and some people get less health care than they need because they lack the resources to pay for it. But many low-income people without insurance *are* served by the health care system, and it is important to compare new proposals with the present system of financing this care in ways that do not show up as a line item of a government budget. A direct subsidy program *will* show up in public expenditures, but much of this apparently extra cost will be offset by the corresponding reduction in hidden costs that in the past were imposed on the private sector.

In addition, the nation's ability to afford direct funding of indigent care depends partly on the willingness to recognize that it may be desirable to redirect policies that now distribute substantial public resources so that support for health care is better targeted to actual need. (For a description of current federal and state programs to assist those with insufficient resources to purchase needed health care services, see Appendix, "Current Policies to Finance Indigent Care," page 102.)

The policy objective for financing indigent care is to assure that no one in America will be denied reasonable access to health care because they are too poor to cover themselves in advance against the possibility of large outlays for health care. Achieving this objective does *not* require a heavy-handed government presence in the marketplace for health insurance. In fact, the CED strategy for health care policy requires that government controls on the price and quantity of services be rolled back.

Moving the government away from cumbersome rate and entry controls will achieve economies in the market. Innovative approaches to health care financing and delivery will be rewarded, and inefficiency will be penalized under a more deregulated, market-oriented system. The saving emerging from a more competitive market is one of several sources of funds for augmenting public support for indigent health care.

STATEMENT OF BASIC PRINCIPLES

CED's vision of an improved health care system is based on a general reliance on market incentives, with government intervention assisting the disadvantaged who would not be able to purchase adequate coverage on their own. In other words, government should allow the market to work and then correct those market outcomes deemed socially unacceptable. Forcing someone to forgo needed health care because he or she is poor is a socially unacceptable outcome. Solving this problem is completely consistent with a market-based approach.

This vision cannot be achieved overnight. But if specific public policy reforms are based on the principles discussed here, we believe that the U.S. health care system can gradually be improved.

- **Government subsidies should be targeted to actual financial need.**

Current health care policy provides subsidies based on categorical groups and personal characteristics rather than actual financial need. This leads government to overcompensate some beneficiaries and to undercompensate others (or exclude them from help entirely). This approach squanders scarce resources by helping some people who could help themselves while leaving legitimate needs unmet.

The desire to target government assistance to those in financial need does not imply that all government programs must include means tests. For social insurance programs such as Medicare and Social Security, it is quite appropriate to provide benefits to all recipients who are eligible by reason of age or disability. But the magnitude of net benefits after taxes can be scaled to ability to pay. This can be accomplished through such means as taxing a greater proportion of the value of government benefits and varying Medicare premium levels with the beneficiary's income.

In an ideal system, people with low incomes would not be denied health care assistance because of their marital status, because their meager incomes come from low-wage jobs rather than welfare, or because they live in a state that has relatively low welfare benefits.

- **Government subsidies should be provided directly to beneficiaries.**

The most efficient use of public resources involves direct subsidies to beneficiaries. Giving aid directly to those who need it fosters the achievements of two objectives simultaneously: First, access to health care is broadened because subsidized patients can choose a health care provider themselves. Second, competition and cost discipline are promoted because providers must vie for subsidized patients by offering high-quality services at competitive prices.

The problem with the indirect approach of giving assistance to service providers is that government aid often turns into a bailout for the inefficient or the ineffective providers. It is difficult to sort out factors that would justify government assistance, such as a disproportionate share of indigent patients, from factors that would not justify subsidies, such as poor management. Government aid to selected providers inevitably underwrites inefficiency even as it relieves cost burdens that are beyond the providers' control. In addition, government aid funneled through service providers does not permit the patient to seek out the best possible value and treatment.

- **The government should offer beneficiaries a choice of health plans and provide incentives for selection of cost effective plans.**

This principle is the public-sector counterpart to the notion that private employers should offer a choice of plans and reward cost-conscious selections. Its advantage is that it fits the pluralistic nature of U.S. health care delivery and financing arrangements. Traditional government policy has operated under the concept that a single plan should be offered to government beneficiaries. Under a more pluralistic approach, a variety of plans and insurance packages could vie for the government's dollar, generating both savings to the public sector in the long run and more options for those being assisted. The government should, of course, screen plans to assure that they provide adequate protection to consumers and should generate sufficient information to facilitate consumers' selections.

- **Some cost sharing for those who can afford it is desirable.**

Cost sharing has been shown to reduce the use of health care services. Generally speaking, cost-conscious decisions are likely to be better than choices made in an environment in which the cost of care is eclipsed by first-dollar coverage.

In fact, first-dollar coverage is rapidly fading from view. Most companies have introduced copayments and deductibles into their health plans. Medicare imposes substantial cost-sharing requirements, and even Medicaid has moved toward limited cost sharing. The challenge is to make some use of cost sharing without going so far as to lead to *underuse* of the health system or imposing financial hardship on low-income patients.

- **Government programs should place greater emphasis on primary care, home care, and prevention and rehabilitation, rather than care in institutional settings.**

As mentioned earlier in this report, private health insurance in America developed and flourished in a way that tied reimbursement to care performed by strictly medical personnel in an institutional or office-based setting. The payment system prevalent in private-sector models and in public programs has favored acute care over prevention and inpatient care over care at home or in an outpatient setting. In recent years, these biases have begun to change as pressure from purchasers has stimulated a movement toward preventive and outpatient care. A substantial amount of surgery is now performed outside of hospitals. This shift has been spurred by both a change in medical opinion and reformed payment practices that have created incentives for less expensive care. In addition, hospice care is now reimbursed by the federal government.

Substantial biases toward more expensive care remain, however, and there is an unfinished reform agenda for the redesign of benefits under public programs. Within limits, it should be possible to achieve economies through encouraging care in lower-cost settings and through early detection and treatment of disease.

There is an important role for managed care to achieve the proper balance between institutional services and home care, and between preventive and curative medicine. Case management and effective discharge planning when a patient leaves a hospital can guide people to care in the most appropriate setting.

- **The principles of effective case management should be built into government programs.**

In order to steer a course between underutilization and overutilization, effective case management is required in the public sector, just as it is the private sector. To guard against overuse, this can involve preadmission screening for hospital stays, second surgical opinions, concurrent stay review, and a primary-care physician's prior authorization of the use of an emergency room or specialists in nonemergency situations. In addition, quality-assurance monitoring is required to make certain that needed care is actually received.

A problem with the greater reimbursement of outpatient services as a cost-containment device is that it usually means paying for services under insurance policies that people were already willing to pay for out of pocket. Once a decision is made to cover certain home or community-based services, it is difficult to limit demand. Indeed, it is not hard to envision a situation in which the savings from patients moved from institutions to outpatient settings are more than offset by the costs of entitling people already receiving care at home.

There are several ways to address this problem. For example, an effective case-management system is needed to develop appropriate criteria for financial support for home care services. This could include requiring a certain degree of disability as a prerequisite for coverage. In addition, the use of coinsurance can help to control outlays.

- **Government programs should provide coverage for catastrophic care.**

Both Medicare and Medicaid lack full protection against the high expenses associated with prolonged or catastrophic illness. As a result, despite all the money that people put into a program such as Medicare (both the payroll taxes they pay when they are working and the substantial cost sharing they shoulder as recipients), Medicare is often not there when they really need it. Benefits should be redesigned to provide a full measure of protection against catastrophic illness.

ESTABLISHING PRIORITIES

What health care services should be included in a subsidized package of benefits? How much is enough? If the government is to redirect subsidies for health care and target them more to need, or if the nation is to give up some other goods and services in order to help the indigent to a greater extent without affecting government aid to the nonpoor, the issue of what constitutes adequate assistance to the poor must be faced. In this type of choice, the perfect can be the enemy of the good. A package that helps with *some* services but not others can be criticized for its omissions, or it can be compared with a situation in which the people in question get no help. Arguments about two-tier medicine are interesting, but for a person with no aid, even a lower tier of help may look attractive.

In moving to help those without any insurance coverage, it may be necessary to choose whether to start at the front end with preventive services and basic primary care, or at the back end, with catastrophic illness protection. A case can be made to start with the front end, where a dollar spent today may save many more dollars tomorrow. This suggests providing public assistance for screening, detection, counseling, and diagnostic services. But it is the really huge outlays that can pauperize a family and that many households simply cannot purchase on their own, whereas some low-income families could pay for basic preventive care. This argues for stop-loss coverage as the first order of business.

One of the troubling aspects of the catastrophic illness approach is that it holds the potential for creating some serious reverse inequities. People with low incomes could gain access to the most expensive technology (e.g., heart or liver transplants) that others with higher incomes could not afford or would become indigent themselves if they tried to purchase. This is surely not to argue the reverse — that such technology should be rationed only to those that can pay — but rather to note that people with little or no financial resources could be entitled to advances in medicine financed by middle- and upper-income taxpayers who themselves might be denied access to the fruits of their investment.

Another consequence could be the underwriting of heroic measures in end-of-life situations at the expense of more routine needs. It is important, therefore, to examine the distribution of health care resources not only across income classes but also across the various types of services. Just as the nation may decide to target limited resources more clearly to financial need, it may decide to target aid within any financial need category based on social and ethical priorities.

APPLICATION OF PRINCIPLES TO GOVERNMENT PROGRAMS

The application of our basic goals and principles for the reform of government programs will gradually transform Medicare and Medicaid.

REFORMING MEDICARE
Medicare lacks a catastrophic-protection feature, fails to relate beneficiary contributions to ability to pay, underestimates the potential insolvency problem under current benefit and tax arrangements, and embroils the government in an ongoing battle with health care providers over the specific prices of individual services.

- **To solve these problems, CED recommends the following reforms:**

  1. **Overhaul the benefit structure to assure full protection for extraordinary health expenses,**

  2. **Treat part of the actuarial value of Medicare benefits as taxable income while relying less on increases in beneficiary cost sharing to make ends meet,**

3. **Merge Part A (hospital costs) and Part B (nonhospital costs) into one fund that is financed more heavily through premiums related to ability to pay,**

4. **Move toward a voucher payment system.**

In essence, Medicare needs new sources of funds for two purposes: to meet the expected revenue shortfall associated with such factors as the aging of the population, and to extend coverage for catastrophic illness. We believe that the best ways to meet these funding requirements are through relating premiums to ability to pay and including a portion of Medicare benefits in taxable income. Both measures are progressive and both avoid taxing the sick while giving those lucky enough to be healthy a free ride. Efforts to address these needs through ever-higher cost sharing would place the financing burden mainly on the sick.

DEFINING CHOICES

Whenever the issue of extending government subsidies for health care comes up, certain questions are always raised: What health care is needed? Should society subsidize preventive care because it seems cost-effective in many cases? Should it cover catastrophic expenses (the back-end coverage rather than front-end preventive outlays) because such outlays can pauperize a family? Should the recipient be able to go to any doctor or hospital, regardless of cost, or should the recipient be led to lower-priced providers in order to conserve public resources?

CED believes that the important question of "How much is enough?" needs to be asked for all members of society, not just those receiving public subsidies. We also believe in a health care system in which some will use dollars in one way and others in a different way. In other words, spending priorities may differ. That is why we favor a choice of health plans, with fixed contributions by employers or government to the various benefit packages. In this way, consumers can select the package of benefits that fits their priorities.

CED believes that it is a mistake for government to specify the precise services that all benefit packages must cover. That is why we oppose the trend toward mandated benefits at the state and federal levels.

We also believe that the types of payment system reforms we advocate will make it easier for people to form their own priorities. By making people more aware of the comparative costs of different types of services, these reforms may help them set priorities.

The important point is to be consistent about the need to make choices, rather than to zero in on the poor while encouraging a free-lunch attitude for the non-poor. The purpose of market-oriented reforms is to help people in all income groups make more informed choices. Our proposed reforms foster this objective.

A little over half of the elderly population has no federal income tax liability and therefore would be unaffected by the taxation of government contributions. To avoid double taxation, Medicare recipients would be taxed only on the portion of benefits funded by other parties — their employers and government. They would not be taxed on the value of their own contributions in the form of the employee's share of Social Security taxes or the Part B premiums they pay as beneficiaries. By taxing senior citizens on the portion of benefits that exceeds what they have contributed to the social insurance system themselves, and using that money to help the neediest citizens in all age groups who are now screened out of public assistance, the nation can move toward generational equity in health care.

The greater reliance on premiums and the taxation of a portion of benefits, coupled with less reliance on higher coinsurance and deductibles, is consistent with our first basic principle of reform: that government benefits should be targeted to financial need. This would also generate the funding, in a progressive way, to foster protection against catastrophic illness. Finally, although cost sharing would be de-emphasized as a revenue raiser, it would not be dropped altogether. If the poor are protected, this approach is consistent with our principle that reasonable amounts of cost sharing play a useful role in health care purchasing decisions.

If the hospital (Part A) and nonhospital (Part B) components of Medicare are merged into one fund, the revenues from the payroll tax would continue to flow into this fund. In addition, both the general revenues of government earmarked for Part B (covering 75 percent of outlays) and beneficiary premium payments (25 percent) would flow into the fund.

In the future, an increase in the Medicare premium should be relied upon to meet the rising cost of the program associated with the aging of the population and technological improvements that lead to higher costs and better health. In general, the actuarial soundness of the fund should not be achieved through higher payroll taxes or general revenues. Relying on the payroll tax is likely to have adverse effects on employment, and the need to control the federal deficit and preserve the contributory nature of Social Security and Medicare rule out greater reliance on general revenues.

It would be possible — and, in our view, desirable — for the relatively affluent elderly and the working-age population (who will be tomorrow's beneficiaries) to share the burden of meeting the higher cost of Medicare. One way to achieve this balance without either raising payroll taxes more than is currently scheduled or raising income tax rates would be to increase excise taxes on alcohol and tobacco. Studies show that consumption of these items varies inversely with their price, and improved health (and perhaps lower outlays for Medicare and other health plans) could be expected as a result.

CED believes that in the long run, the solution to the problem of how Medicare should pay the providers of health services is the adoption of a voucher system. Under this arrangement, Medicare beneficiaries would be given vouchers to purchase any qualified health plan operating in their area. Medicare would offer a cash rebate to beneficiaries who select a plan with a premium below the voucher amount. Those choosing a plan with a premium above the voucher amount would pay the difference themselves.

Voucher amounts could vary according to the age and sex of the enrollee, and at least during a transitional period, the value of the voucher might vary according to the relative medical spending in the region. Vouchers would permit and encourage the beneficiaries to participate in new types of health plans. These plans would have more opportunities to market their services to enrollees, and cost savings over the long run could be expected to emerge from the broader competition for Medicare's caseload.

However, there are some possible negative effects of vouchers, including a threat of adverse and preferred risk selection that could result in a transfer of costs from low users of the system to high users. Some critics fear that vouchers would erode the entitlement nature of Medicare and make it too easy to cut spending for the program. Moreover, vouchers will not save money overnight; the potential economies will unfold only over an extended period of time.

The advantage of a voucher is that it phases the government out of the role of setting prices for health services. Government can never effectively substitute for the private market in the proper determination of the relative prices of various goods and services. This is as true in health care as it is in the steel or the petroleum industries. A voucher system would turn the function of price setting and the details of program management over to private-sector managers.

The voucher approach would breathe life into two of the basic principles of reform: fostering a choice of plans with incentives to beneficiaries to select cost-effective coverage and providing subsidies directly to individuals who qualify for government assistance.

SPECIFIC PROGRAM FEATURES AND REFORMS

The long-range, wholesale reform of Medicare may take years to develop and will be difficult to achieve. Therefore, it may be necessary to adopt some shorter-term, less comprehensive, but still basic reforms that are consistent with the ultimate reform objective.

The present Medicare benefit structure does not provide adequate protection against extended and very expensive illnesses. After a patient pays a deductible equivalent to the average cost of one night in a hospital (currently $520), the next fifty-nine days are covered in full. Between the sixtieth and ninetieth days of a long-term stay, Medicare charges the patient one-fourth of the daily bill (an average of $130). After the ninetieth day, this charge rises to half the bill. Moreover, patients are allotted a lifetime reserve to cover extraordinary hospital costs; when that reserve is exhausted, Medicare pays no portion of the bill. Although the proportion of Medicare beneficiaries who are in a hospital this long is very small, the financial hardship for those people is severe.

An elderly person might also face huge doctor bills without reaching a limit on out-of-pocket outlays. Medicare covers 80 percent of what it deems the allowable physician's fee, leaving the patient responsible for the remaining 20 percent. If physicians agree to hold their fees to the level allowed by Medicare, a process called *accepting assignment*, they cannot bill the patient for any amount in excess of this level. (Medicare now offers a variety of incentives for doctors to accept assignment.) But physicians have the right to refuse assignment; and if they do, they can bill the patient for the amount of their charge in excess of the Medicare payment. If a person has major surgery and is faced with the uncovered portions of the surgeon's bill and the bills of several consulting physicians, these charges can mount up rapidly. For the very poor elderly, Medicaid may pay the copayments and deductibles, but people a little over the eligibility threshold for this Medicare-Medicaid *dual eligibility* can face uncovered charges that can be beyond their ability to pay.

Finally, Medicare covers very little in the way of long-term care outside of the hospital. Benefits cover only 100 days in a skilled nursing facility, and patients make a sizable copayment between the twentieth and hundredth days. Moreover, Medicare does not cover any custodial care received at home (neither does Medicaid). Thus, an elderly person who is chronically disabled and at home typically has to finance required services such as around-the-clock nurses on an out-of-pocket basis regardless of how modest his or her means may be. Again, Medicare — a $70 billion program — is sometimes not there when it is most needed.

- **CED recommends that a stop-loss provision be built into Medicare in a revenue-neutral way to cover outlays for such basic benefits as hospitalization, physician's fees, X rays, and laboratory tests. After beneficiaries make out-of-pocket outlays of a given amount in any one year, they would not have to make further payments.**

Administrative simplicity would suggest that the stop-loss amount be fixed for all beneficiaries (e.g., $3,000) and updated annually. However, there are wide variations in the Medicare population's ability to pay. Therefore, we recommend that the stop-loss amount be related to a household's income. This could be accomplished through a schedule with a few brackets of payment limits corresponding to income brackets or through setting the limit at some percentage of the previous year's adjusted gross income (say, 15 percent).

The current Medicare program favors acute health care over long-term care. Coverage for long-term care occurs at the front end of need (Medicare covers the first 100 days in a skilled nursing facility) and is tied to institutional care. One approach to reducing the current imbalance would be to set a somewhat higher stop-loss amount for acute care (e.g., $5,000 instead of $2,000 to $3,000) and extend a little more protection for long-term care. The latter could be accomplished if Medicare served a reinsurance function that afforded some limit to the losses of private insurers of long-term care.

If the plan proposed by U.S. Secretary of Health and Human Services Bowen were modified to provide a range of stop-loss amounts scaled to income (e.g., from $1,500 per year to $5,000 per year) and the same additional Part B premium envisioned by Bowen were collected ($4.92 per month), some funds would be freed up for long-term care. If additional revenues were generated through the taxation of Medicare benefits, the combined revenue gain could permit a stop-loss provision to be built into Medicare for long-term care. This stop-loss would have to be set at a rather high level (e.g., $75,000 or $100,000). Alternatively, Medicare could reinsure private long-term care policies for outlays above such limits.

This approach would be preferable to adding government coverage at the front end of long-term care; the government should not intercede and insure all kinds of chronic care needs, and people should be encouraged to set aside their own resources or obtain private insurance for such needs. If government rearranged its coverage to provide more of a protective umbrella for truly catastrophic events (regardless of whether they were called acute or long-term), the role of private insurance in the acute care sector would be preserved and the role of private insurance for long-term care would be invigorated.

Some notes of caution must be sounded here: First although catastrophic illness insurance, as might be accomplished through a stop-loss provision, would rationalize the Medicare benefit structure and avert huge financial losses for some consumers, it could lead to a situation in which there was little or no check on the development or application of new technology to treat critically or terminally ill patients. In effect, a stop-loss removes the price mechanism as a factor in decisions at the margin after the stop-loss is exceeded.

If this occurs, it may be necessary to consider other ways to ration the use of resources in end-of-life or heroic intervention situations. Without prices to allocate resources, it may be necessary *either* to place some administrative limits on use *or* to understand that providers and the families of patients are being given a blank check.

There are, of course, checks on unrestrained use of resources even under a stop-loss structure: Medicare has converted from a reimbursement system based on actual costs to a system of prospectively set limits for hospital payments. Under the new DRG system, the money runs out at some point because the hospital is getting paid on the basis of normal utilization of services for each illness. Of course, some variation is expected, but if a case becomes too costly, the hospital will be losing money for each additional service unless the patient's family can pay.

Moreover, there is increasing uneasiness in the United States today about the desirability of limitless care in hopeless medical situations. Although personal and family views differ on this, as is desirable in a free society, the growing interest in living wills reflects a desire to balance the goal of preserving life at all cost with the goal of preserving the dignity of life.

Second, many Medicare beneficiaries are covered today for these extensive hospital stays beyond sixty days by private insurance, or so-called Medigap policies. But about a third of the elderly do not have such policies, and it has been argued that Medicare could fill this need more efficiently than private insurance. In our view, there is room for both public and private insurance to cover catastrophic health expenses. Our point here is not to stipulate a precise stop-loss figure or an exact line delineating government and private-sector roles, but rather to argue for a basic redesign of Medicare coverage that is consistent with the concept of full protection for all senior citizens against unusually high medical expenses.

ENCOURAGING PREVENTION AND OUTPATIENT CARE

Specific steps should be taken to correct some of the features of Medicare that discourage preventive care and encourage the use of high-cost inpatient facilities where more reasonably priced, safe, and effective alternatives exist. For example, the fact that Medicare does not cover most of the charges associated with a regular physical examination may discourage the regular annual checkup, reducing opportunities to detect health problems early. Also, the low cap of $250 per year on outpatient visits for mental health services coupled with up to *190* days of coverage for inpatient hospital care for mental health may encourage the use of relatively more expensive hospital care. Many surgical procedures can be done safely on an outpatient basis, and the Medicare benefit structure should further encourage the use of such outpatient surgery.

- **CED recommends that Medicare benefits be redesigned in a budget-neutral way to encourage preventive health care and care in outpatient or community settings where such care can be safely substituted for inpatient hospital care.**

PAYMENT SYSTEM REFORMS

In 1983, Medicare instituted the DRG system of prospective payments, establishing fixed rates of reimbursement for 467 categories of illness. This new system is a vast improvement over the cost-based reimbursement approach that simply ratified and underwrote cost escalation. Under the new system, hospitals that hold costs below the DRG payment rates may keep the difference, but hospitals whose costs exceed the rates must absorb the difference. Thus, the new system rewards hospitals that prudently manage their resources and penalizes profligacy.

However, the DRG system raises a number of problems. Ultimately, of course, we believe it should be a stepping-stone to a voucher plan. The DRG system plunges the government into setting prices (which would not be the case under a voucher plan) and these prices are based on average costs. This vestige of the regulated-price model based on average cost is less efficient than pricing decisions made by individual providers on the basis of marginal costs.

The new system at least has the virtue of pricing an episode of illness rather than each individual service, thereby encouraging hospitals to use and price such services economically. But government will always run behind the private sector in its ability to adjust its prices to a rapidly changing environment. Adjustments for quality improvement and technological change will be technically difficult to arrive at and highly vulnerable to political pressures. Given the ongoing pressure of the federal deficit, there will be a temptation to bypass needed increases in DRG prices in order to hold down federal outlays. Of course, this same pressure might hold the value of a voucher below the appropriate level.

Moreover, DRGs are still somewhat incomplete as a cost control measure because they set a prospective rate once a patient is in a hospital but do not offer incentives for physicians to be more cost-conscious about hospitalizing patients in the first place.

The federal government has also developed a new approach to paying HMOs and other so-called *competitive medical plans (CMPs)*. Qualifying HMOs and CMPs receive 95 percent of the adjusted average per capita cost in each area of the country for each enrolled recipient. The federal government shares the savings generated by such plans with beneficiaries. If, for example, a plan can serve enrollees for 80 percent of the average cost in its area, the government, by paying 95 percent, saves 5 percent of what it would otherwise pay, and the plan must pass on the additional 15 percentage points of savings (payments based on 95 percent of the average less its costs that are 80 percent of that average) to the enrollee in the form of additional benefits. Plans may not offer cash rebates, however, or plough back the savings into uses such as recruitment of new medical staff or the purchases of new equipment. They may help beneficiaries in one way only: offering added benefits.

Both approaches — DRGs and HMO/CMP risk-sharing arrangements — could be stepping-stones to a voucher system. To move this process along and improve the new approaches, CED recommends the following steps:

- **Update DRGs fairly and fully for inflation and technological change.**

- **Reimburse capital costs on a basis that reflects the replacement cost of capital rather than using some arbitrary cap or ceiling.**

- **Move the DRG program toward a more comprehensive payment that includes incentives for avoiding unnecessary hospitalization.**

- **Broaden the options open to HMOs and CMPs with regard to the use of savings generated by lower costs. Allow cash rebates and ploughbacks that promise to improve the quality of care over time.**

- **Relax the definition of HMOs and other qualifying plans under Medicare to include other innovative health plans with cost-saving potential such as preferred provider plans.**

PHYSICIAN PAYMENT REFORMS

The current structure of Medicare's payment system for physicians is a model of adverse incentives. It has hardly been changed since the program began two decades ago. Medicare pays 80 percent of allowable charges after the beneficiary has paid a $75 deductible. Allowed charges are based on the lowest of three screens: (1) the physician's billed charge, (2) the physician's customary charge, (3) the prevailing charge in the community, defined as the seventy-fifth percentile of customary charges for the same service. The permissible rise in the prevailing charge has been limited since the early 1970s to the annual rate of increase in the Medicare Economic Index, a measure of physician costs.

This system sends all the wrong signals to physicians. The unit of payment, individual services, encourages unnecessary tests and procedures. The basis for the level of payment, current charges, encourages physicians to keep charges high. The basis for differences in charges for different services, historical relationships, favors the provision of procedures in high-cost inpatient settings over lower-cost outpatient settings. And the basis for pricing new services, initial charges, is never modified; consequently, productivity improvements are not shared by Medicare.

Payment reform options can be placed on a continuum related to the degree to which services are combined (bundled) for payment purposes. The lowest level of bundling is the individual service unit. The highest level is a full capitation model (payment per capita over a specified period). In between is a payment-by-diagnosis (DRG-type) approach.

Even if no bundling is undertaken, it would be possible to convert Medicare physician payment under the current approach to a fee-schedule basis. Some limits would be set according to a schedule of fees rather than riding up as physicians raise their charges.

Each of these options has advantages and disadvantages, but they are all superior to the current system of *customary, prevailing, and reasonable (CPR)* fee reimbursement. Along this continuum, control over costs becomes increasingly comprehensive. However, some risks associated with more fully capitated approaches are enlarged.

Under a merged Part A, Part B program and a voucher plan, individual service pricing by government would end. Until this occurs, however, **CED recommends that the federal government move away from the traditional CPR physician payment system. The government should experiment with and explore the potential of new arrangements such as fee schedules, relative-value scales, DRGs, and capitation and should move toward the most cost-effective alternative to the present system.**

REFORMING MEDICAID

There are four major problems with current government policy toward indigent care: (1) Eligibility for government assistance is tied to arbitrary welfare rules that screen many poor people out of coverage. (2) Extremely low government payment rates discourage provider participation in the Medicaid program. (3) Medicaid offers poor incentives for providers and patients to be cost-conscious in the use of health care resources. (4) Inadequate attention is paid to prevention and primary care.

COST CONTROL AND AVOIDING FALSE ECONOMIES

The traditional approach to cost control under Medicaid actually entrenched inefficiency and discouraged participation in the program by doctors and other providers. Limits on allowable increases in hospital charges involved applying the same percentage increases in revenues to all hospitals, regardless of their relative costs. Complex formulas and revenue caps failed to reward the innovative, cost-conscious provider. Along with controls on entry into the hospital industry in the form of certificate-of-need regulation, this system of reimbursement resembled the public utility regulation model of cost control. There is considerable evidence that this approach has failed to check the rapid rise in health care costs.[1]

Medicaid also tried to control costs by freezing fee levels for physicians. Many states have not raised fees for doctors under Medicaid for up to a decade, and rates as low as $7 to $10 for an office visit have been common in recent years, leading to a decrease in physician participation in Medicaid.[2]

At the same time that Medicaid programs pushed down allowable fees and charges, they generally turned their backs on the *quantity* of health services used. Thus, the way to prosper while serving Medicaid patients was to set up so-called *Medicaid mills*, running thousands of patients through batteries of tests and procedures.

The combination of low reimbursement rates and the allowance of open-ended use of the system designed to give low income households maximum freedom of choice backfired. In many areas this freedom became hypothetical as primary-care doctors (internists, pediatricians, obstetricians) withdrew from participation. Patients have often used the emergency room or the outpatient clinic of a hospital as their point of entry into the system, seeking care much later than was appropriate and obtaining it in an unnecessarily high-cost setting.

Many states are now turning to prospective budgeting and are experimenting with new and more promising systems of managed care that change the incentives for both beneficiaries and providers. These include:

- *Designating a doctor or other health care provider to serve as a patient's case manager and point of entry to the system*. The case manager channels the patient to care in the most appropriate setting and must authorize nonemergency referrals to specialists and hospitalization. Patients receive care from a provider who is familiar with his or her medical history and who also tends to provide more preventive care.

- *Giving providers more financial incentives to participate and to use resources prudently*. Per unit prices are set a little closer to market levels, but the providers share in the risk of total cost levels. If utilization is held down to normal levels, the physicians' reimbursement would be higher than if utilization is excessive.

- *Providing incentives for long-term care at home or in the community (where possible).* This takes the place of the traditional model that skews public assistance heavily toward long-term care in an institution.

LONG-TERM REFORM

The Medicaid program should be reformed to improve its fairness and to incorporate more efficient and effective methods of paying for services.

The long-term objective for Medicaid reform is to achieve universal coverage for health services while promoting a more competitive health care market and minimizing government control. We believe this can best be achieved through replacing the current program with a set of refundable federal tax credits. These credits would be set at a level that would permit people to pay the premium for basic health insurance. In other words, the government would help the poor buy into the private health insurance system.

Eligibility for this credit would be uncoupled from the welfare system and would be based on financial need alone. In fact, as proposed by Professor Alain Enthoven of Stanford University, this tax credit could be made completely universal, replacing the current system of tax preferences involving the unlimited exclusion by employees of employer contributions to health insurance.[3]

Under the approach developed by Enthoven, the value of the subsidy would vary with such factors as age and sex, and it would be updated annually.

The approach ties in with and reinforces several of our basic principles. First, subsidies are paid directly to individuals, not through providers. Second, the fixed-dollar limit on these subsidies (at any given time) would promote a more competitive marketplace for insurance. Third, the refundable credits would be much more clearly related to financial need than the current patchwork system, with all of its obvious inequities.

An alternative to a system of universal tax credits replacing both the current open-ended tax preferences and Medicaid is a sliding-scale voucher program. Under this approach, Medicaid would be converted to a voucher, and the government would make a payment to a private health plan chosen by the beneficiary. A variety of health plans, including the Blues, commercial insurance policies, PPOs, and HMOs, would compete for the government's subsidy. This voucher approach would not necessarily have to be coupled with the substitution of fixed tax credits for the current open-ended tax exclusion enjoyed by the working population.

A central feature of the voucher approach would be a sliding-scale government contribution to the plan, based on the beneficiary's income. Poor people would have the full amount of the voucher paid by government. (Nominal cost sharing, such as $3 for an office visit to a doctor and $1 for a prescription, could be allowed to discourage unnecessary use of health services.) For those with incomes in the near-poor range, the government's contribution would drop, and the beneficiary would have to contribute to the total voucher cost. The amount that the near-poor contribute would need to be significant in order to avert a situation in which people would drop private coverage (or employers would drop them from company plans) in order to transfer to the subsidized program.

The advantage of the sliding-scale phaseout of a voucher plan is that it could correct the *notch problems* associated with the Medicaid program. Notch problems arise when an extra dollar of earnings causes a household to lose eligibility for public assistance. With no gradual phase-down in benefits, households are in danger of falling over the cliff if they exert extra effort in the labor market.

Yet another alternative is a federal block grant to states to use in broadening coverage to those poor households ineligible for Medicaid. This approach would keep Medicaid but fuse onto it a block grant to cover such groups as the working poor in two-parent families. To avert the problem of a disincentive for private coverage, the level of this grant could be set to provide only catastrophic-illness coverage.

INTERIM CHANGES CONSISTENT WITH LONG-TERM REFORM

A number of interim steps can be taken to improve and rationalize the current welfare-Medicaid system.

States establish need standards for determining AFDC and Medicaid eligibility. The *need standard* is the amount of money considered necessary for a family to meet subsistence needs. A household is eligible today for AFDC only if its gross income is less than 185 percent of the need standard in the state.

At first glance, this might seem generous. But most state need standards are well below the federal poverty line. For example, in Kentucky, which has the lowest need standard in the country, the standard for a family of four in 1986 was $246 a month, or $2,952 a year. This is less than one-third of the federal poverty line. A household in Kentucky could have 185 percent of this state need standard and still have only $5,461 in annual income, which is less than half of the poverty line for a family of four. Thus, in Kentucky, any four-person household with a gross income that exceeds about half of the federal poverty line is screened out of AFDC and therefore Medicaid for having too much gross income.

Of course, need standards vary greatly from state to state. For example, in Oklahoma, the standard was $349 a month in 1986 for a family of four, or $4,188 per year. A household in Oklahoma could have up to $7,748 in annual income (about three-fourths of the poverty-line income) and qualify for AFDC. The cutoff line in Wisconsin, where the monthly need standard for a family of four is $749, is $16,627. Thus, a four-person household in Wisconsin could have a gross income of $16,000 and still slip under the AFDC gross income limit. This is three times as high as the limit in Kentucky.

These figures illustrate the dramatic regional differences in the AFDC-Medicaid complex. Some families with half of the poverty line income are screened out while other households with one and a half times the poverty line are eligible.

In fact, AFDC eligibility is really even more stringent than these numbers suggest. In addition to the 185 percent limit on gross income, AFDC also requires countable income to be less than a state's payment standard, which is the maximum benefit a state will actually pay. States may set the payment standard at some fraction of their own need standards. Thus, although need standards are often below the poverty line, payment standards are often even less. For example, in Alabama, the 1986 AFDC payment standard (maximum benefits) was set at $147 a month for a family of four, or $1,764 a year. This amount is only about one-sixth of the federal poverty line. Families with higher incomes are ineligible for AFDC and will therefore typically also be denied Medicaid.

We do not mean to suggest that benefit levels in public assistance programs should be uniform across geographic areas. In fact, differences in the cost of living and in the cost of medical services might justify some regional variation in benefits. (Some observers, however, would caution against fully underwriting geographic differences in medical costs.) Moreover, a case can be made for allowing states some flexibility in the generosity of their public assistance benefits. Clearly, however, the magnitude of the differences in Medicaid eligibility standards and payment levels is indefensible. When the criteria employed by some states are three times as stringent as those used in other states, a sense of basic fairness is violated.

- **CED recommends that the federal government establish a floor on Aid to Families with Dependent Children benefits at a level that assures at least the poorest of the poor eligibility for Medicaid.**

This minimum standard could be set at some level such as one-half, two-thirds, or three-fourths of the federal poverty line. States could be required to bring their AFDC benefits into line with such a floor in order to receive federal matching money under AFDC and Medicaid. Further incentives for raising the eligibility standard toward the poverty line could be provided by increasing the federal matching rate as states raise the threshold. Under this arrangement, states would get no matching federal dollars until they reached the minimum. Once the minimum was reached, they would get a federal match on all outlays; and above the minimum, this match might be increased.

A 1985 study prepared for the House Ways and Means Committee by the Congressional Research Service and the Congressional Budget Office provided cost estimates for a package of four proposals designed to extend basic public assistance to many of the impoverished households now excluded from help:[4]

- Mandate a minimum benefit level.

- Extend benefits to two-parent families.

- Increase allowable deductions from income.

- Liberalize asset restrictions.

- Reduce states' financing shares for increases in AFDC benefits.

More specifically, the package involves setting AFDC and food stamp benefits so that the combination would equal 65 percent of the poverty income guidelines for each family size. In 1986, the AFDC minimum benefit for a family of three would be $396 under this formula, with food stamps at a minimum of $132.[5]

The old "$30 and a third" work incentive that was largely scrapped in 1981 (the "disregard" of one-third of earnings was limited to only four months of work) would be reinstated at a level of $50 plus one-fourth of earnings. The optional portion of AFDC for two-parent households with one parent either unemployed or working 100 hours or less per month (Aid to Families with Dependent Children-Unemployed Parent, or AFDC-U) would become mandatory for all states. Deductions for child care and work expenses would be raised, and the asset test would be increased to a maximum of $2,250 (from $1,000).

The estimated net cost of this proposal in fiscal 1986 was $5.3 billion. The price tag would more than double over five years to a projected $11.3 billion in fiscal 1990. Of the $5.3 billion, the federal government would pay $3.3 billion and states $2.0 billion.[6]

A proposal by U.S. Senator Daniel Evans would set the benefit floor (including both AFDC cash benefits and the cash value of food stamps) at 50 percent of the federal poverty line initially and then raise it in annual increments of 2 percentage points until it reached 62 percent. The federal government would pay 90 percent of the value of this grant up to the 62 percent floor. Above the floor, states would be reimbursed by the federal government at current, lower rates.

The Evans plan also mandates the AFDC-U program. This proposal would raise federal AFDC costs by $3.5 to $4 billion in fiscal 1988. However, most of this cost is offset by a reduction in state outlays that is almost as great. This trade-off would result from the very high federal matching rate (90 percent) designed to pull up benefit levels in the very low-benefit states. Although this portion of the proposal mainly trades federal for state spending, the federal government would have to devise offsetting budget policies to prevent the added $3.5 to $4.0 billion from adding to the deficit. The Evans proposal details a set of expenditure cuts that would make the floor on AFDC and other proposed reforms budget neutral.

- **CED recommends that whatever the proportion of the poverty line established as a cash-assistance floor, more people who fall between the line of eligibility for cash assistance and the federal poverty line should be qualified to receive Medicaid.**

Establishing a national floor on AFDC benefits would automatically bring health care coverage to many poor households in states that now have very restrictive AFDC eligibility criteria. This would occur because AFDC opens the door to Medicaid. But if this national floor is below the poverty line, there will still be poor households without health coverage.

Many of the uninsured are working at low-wage jobs. It is not necessary to extend Medicaid to all of these workers if a private-sector solution can be worked out that assures them coverage. The important point to stress is that public coverage for workers should not compete with private coverage or encourage firms that do provide insurance to drop that coverage and place the workers on Medicaid. If a voucher covering the equivalent of only catastrophic expense protection with high copayments and deductibles were available for workers without private insurance, there would be a fall-back or safety net for the working poor, and yet they would still be better off with a more comprehensive, regular insurance policy. This would provide protection without encouraging firms to ask workers to switch over to Medicaid.

Medicaid extension, however, is still needed, particularly to cover groups such as unemployed heads of households and other poor people without jobs who are screened out of public insurance as a result of arbitrary categorical eligibility criteria. And, it is certainly feasible to cover some of the working poor publicly while others receive employer-provided protection.

In addition, many elderly and disabled people whose incomes are below the poverty line do not receive Medicaid. In fact, only about a third of the elderly poor receive Medicaid, which pays for the copayments and deductibles under Medicare as well as providing greater coverage for long-term care than Medicare offers.

The advantage of uncoupling health care assistance from cash assistance is that health care coverage may be much more important to low-income people than the relatively small amount of cash assistance for which they would qualify. For example, if a household had three-fourths of a poverty-level income, its cash benefits would be rather small if it qualifies for AFDC. Yet, this family could be easily wiped out by any health expenses other than the most routine outlays. This measure would afford such households protection even as the debate about what to do with the basic welfare system continues and even if the decision is to keep it as it is.

The Evans proposal would extend publicly funded health care coverage to children under five years old (rising in stages a year at a time to age eleven), to all pregnant women, to the elderly who are poor but not receiving Supplemental Security Income (SSI) benefits, and to people a little above the welfare eligibility threshold who are made poor by paying large medical bills. These changes would add about $4.2 billion to fiscal 1988 federal outlays, which would be only partially offset by reductions in state expenditures for Medicaid. Thus, a rough estimate of the total additional federal cost of setting a floor on cash-assistance benefits and assuring health coverage to most groups left out of the cash-assistance system (AFDC plus Medicaid) would be about $8 billion in FY 1988. State outlays would fall by about half this amount.

- **While waiting for fundamental reforms in financing indigent health care, CED supports state government efforts to fill in some of the gaps in the welfare-Medicaid system.**

Indigent care pools funded by state, county, and private-sector contributions are channeling resources to providers who have a disproportionately high share of uncompensated health care. The approach adopted in South Carolina (see "The South Carolina Approach," page 106) provides a good model. It expands Medicaid coverage, establishes an indigent care risk pool for the non-Medicaid poor, and devises reforms in the payment systems to foster greater efficiency. Subsidizing certain providers is a second-best solution, but it is preferable to no action at all.

- **The Medicaid dollar should be stretched farther through better systems of paying providers.**

The government should abandon price controls and turn to incentives that reward cost-effective health plans. Effective cost management under primary-care network arrangements offers physicians incentives to participate in Medicaid and to use resources in a cost-conscious manner. When unnecessary use of services is controlled, resources are freed to offer physicians a reasonable fee for their services. But additional resources can also be used to extend coverage or at least to avoid further cutbacks in services covered under Medicaid. Physicians should share a portion of the risk as well as a portion of the rewards of cost-effective care.

In addition to these risk-sharing arrangements with doctors and prospective payments for hospitals, states are also beginning to encourage alternatives to hospital and nursing home care through channeling long-term care patients to the most appropriate setting.

It is hard to calculate the savings arising from a greater reliance on managed care under Medicaid. But these savings will gradually emerge and can help to meet the costs of our proposals for filling in some of the cracks in the health-related social protection system.

REGULATORY REFORM

The government should promote rather than restrict entry into health care markets and should encourage choices among health plans that offer consumers various combinations of benefits at varying costs. Opportunities to substitute lower-cost for higher-cost services should be fostered in ways that are consistent with standards that protect public safety and promote high-quality care.

To achieve these essential ingredients of a competitive market, CED recommends the following steps:

- **De-emphasize certificate-of-need restrictions and government planning decisions governing resource allocation in health care.**

- **Avoid public mandates requiring employers or insurance companies to include specified benefits in every health plan.**

- **Ease restrictions that limit the access of certain types of professionals, such as nurse midwives, to hospital staffs or other privileges. While we favor opening up institutions to a greater variety of professionals, we oppose mandating insurance coverage of their services.**

- **Assure that conditions of participation in programs such as Medicare do not preserve anachronistic or unnecessary requirements on service providers.**

- **Use existing antitrust law to assure that industry reconfigurations and behavior are consistent with a competitive marketplace.**

FINANCING COMMITMENTS

- **CED recommends that the government develop a system of paying for indigent care that ends the arbitrary discrimination against large segments of the population. We believe that these commitments should be fully financed. It would be a mistake to rely on additions to the federal deficit to underwrite new commitments to those in need. To do so would simply be to relieve one hardship while contributing to others.**

CED has taken a firm position regarding the desirability of lower marginal tax rates. Where it is possible and equitable, we believe that it would be preferable to finance new public-sector commitments through a broader tax base or through a reduction in public expenditures that does not create serious financial hardship for beneficiaries.

A good starting point in the effort to tighten the basic safety net involves more complete taxation of government benefits than now occurs. Without changing benefits under federal programs such as Social Security and Medicare, we could subject such benefits more fully to taxation. This would raise revenues without increasing the burden on lower-income senior citizens.

One option for funding indigent care would be to tax the amount of Social Security benefits that exceeds total contributions by employees. This is consistent with private pension practices. If 85 percent of benefits were taxed instead of the current rate of 50 percent (above certain thresholds), the tax treatment of Social Security benefits would approximate the corresponding tax treatment of private pensions. The Congressional Budget Office estimates that the taxation of 85 percent of Social Security benefits would generate $4.6 billion in 1988 and $74.0 billion over 1988-1992 period.

These estimates reflect combining two steps: taxing 85 percent of benefits instead of the current 50 percent and eliminating the current thresholds of $32,000 for couples and $25,000 for individuals. Thus, more people would be subjected to a tax and a larger proportion of benefits would be taxed. If these thresholds were not eliminated, but lowered from current levels to $18,000 and $12,000 for joint and single returns, respectively, the cumulative five-year revenue gain would be $39.5 billion instead of $74.0 billion if 85 percent of benefits were taxed. If the thresholds were lowered in this way, but 50 percent of benefits were taxed, as at present, the five-year revenue gain is estimated by CBO to be $14.2 billion.[7]

Another option is to include part of the actuarial value of Medicare in taxable income. It is vital to avoid double taxation in this area, too. This can be done by taxing only 50 percent of the value of Part A benefits and 75 percent of the value of Part B benefits. These amounts reflect the employer's contributions to hospital benefits (Part A) and the government's contributions to expenses for physician's fees, laboratory tests, equipment and the like (Part B). The retiree would not be taxed on his or her contributions to Medicare — the half of the payroll tax (earmarked for Part A) the retiree paid while working or one-fourth of the Part B cost that this retiree pays in the form of an insurance premium.

If part of the value of Medicare benefits were included in taxable income in a way that avoids double taxation, this would, according to CBO estimates, raise $0.7 billion in 1988. This estimate assumes that 50 percent of hospital insurance (Part A of Medicare) benefits and 75 percent of Part B benefits are taxed, and that the current Social Security tax thresholds are kept intact and also applied to Medicare. The five-year (1988-1992) cumulative revenue increase from taxing the value of Medicare benefits in this way is estimated at $14.0 billion. If we assume that the Social Security tax thresholds are eliminated and that all income is taxable with the proportion of Medicare benefits taxed, as just described, the revenue estimates rise to $1.4 billion in 1988 and to $25.6 billion over the period.[8]

The revenues collected through additional taxation of government social insurance benefits would flow into the Social Security trust funds. The outlays needed to strengthen the safety net would involve general revenues. In our view, however, if offsetting steps are taken that are budget-neutral when the entire federal budget — including trust funds — is taken into account, the total package is fiscally responsible.[9]

We believe that the cost of providing health care benefits cannot be borne entirely by the elderly; the working-age population should share the burden. One option for accomplishing this is the partial taxation of employee health insurance benefits. Federal tax policy has encouraged both the demand for health services and the construction of facilities to meet that demand. Allowing employees to exclude the full amount of employer contributions to health insurance from taxable income has led to the spread and enrichment of employee group health insurance.

This development has provided a broad private network of protection that has increased access to health care for millions of Americans, and by doing this through the workplace, has offered an alternative to the national health insurance plans featured in many other countries. Moreover, the deductibility of health care outlays above some threshold has insulated people with serious illness from some of the attendant financial hardships. The tax treatment of hospital construction financing helped assure access to care in various communities previously under-served and, along the way, helped to fund indigent care through the charity care obligation in the Hill-Burton program.

Many of the conditions that originally motivated these tax preferences — widespread inadequate coverage of the working population, insufficient capacity in the hospital sector, etc. — have now changed. Most workers now have health coverage (though a disturbing number of low-wage workers do not) and health facilities are now *over-built* rather than in short supply.

Some observers believe that the favorable tax treatment of health insurance leads to inefficiency in health insurance markets, while others believe that such inefficiency is being wrung out of the health care system by more aggressive and effective cost-management techniques. Some believe that tax preferences for employee health insurance reflect poor targeting of government assistance. Others assert that such tax preferences are by no means equivalent to direct expenditure programs and are deserved by workers who are being taxed to help the disadvantaged as well as to provide for their own retirement.

There are merits to both sides of this controversy. We believe, however, that a ceiling on this tax preference would help to strengthen the trend toward cost discipline in the health insurance market. It will encourage employers who have not yet acted to redesign their health plans or offer more choice of plans, with incentives for workers to select a cost-effective plan, to take such steps. Moreover, by bringing working-age people into the financing of coverage extensions along with senior citizens whose benefits would be taxed, it fosters a sense of intergenerational sharing. And it would raise additional revenue that could help finance the cost of the reforms proposed here.

There are some objections to this proposal because of the administrative difficulties of determining the value of benefits to be included in taxable income. This could be a particular problem for firms with operations in several regions of the country. Additional problems would arise from borderline decisions about what is actually included in the benefits package. A number of activities engaged in by companies that are often not part of a health plan nonetheless may affect health costs. For example, a firm may offer (or mandate) annual physical examinations that are not included in the benefit package but affect health status and long-run health expenditures. Therefore, clearly delineating what is included in a health plan in order to arrive at an actuarial value for imputing potential tax liability could be a problem under a tax-cap policy.

Our point here is that a ceiling on tax preferences related to group health insurance should be considered as an important financing option for extending health insurance to the uncovered poor. The ceiling should be placed on the employee's exclusion of the employer contribution to health insurance.

The ceiling on the amount of an employer's contribution that can be excluded from an employee's taxable income should be set at a relatively high level so that it affects mainly people with very comprehensive insurance coverage. In 1987, for example, a ceiling of about $200 a month would impose little or no additional taxes on most workers with standard health insurance plans. The ceiling could be initially set so that the majority of workers face no added tax bite while those who do pay extra taxes are subjected to a reasonable increase (e.g., $200 to $300 a year). The important point is not to use this measure as a major revenue raiser in the first year but to establish the principle that at the margin, people who opt for a more expensive plan should contribute a little bit to the extra cost.

One proposal to limit the exclusion would treat as taxable income any employer contributions to health insurance that exceed $200 a month for family health insurance policies and $80 a month for individual policies (in 1988 dollars), with these amounts indexed to reflect inflation. This step would raise an estimated $3.2 billion in federal revenues in 1988 (including income and payroll tax revenue increases). The annual total revenue increase would grow to $10.0 billion in 1992, and the cumulative five-year addition to federal revenues (1988-1992) would be $34.3 billion, of which $22.2 billion represents added federal income taxes and $12.1 billion represents greater payroll tax revenue.[10]

Another option for financing additional health care coverage is an increase in excise taxes. In particular, a higher tax on alcohol and cigarettes would generate revenues at the same time as it would improve the health of the population by discouraging the consumption of these substances.

Finally, it would be possible to make room for additional outlays for extending publicly funded health insurance by scaling back other government expenditures. Everyone has his or her favorite candidates, and each program has its own advocates. Some would cut back national defense outlays; others would look to farm subsidies, transportation subsidies, or urban redevelopment programs. Rather than pass judgment on such matters, we seek to establish the principle that the nation *could* afford additional outlays if it wishes to make basic health coverage for the poor a priority. It is necessary to proceed in a fashion that does not either ignore the cost or transfer the cost to our children through irresponsible fiscal policies. In one way or another, the nation must bring its commitments and its available resources into line.

These recommendations, taken together, reflect a new vision of the government role in health care in the United States. The government should do what it is *well suited to do* — provide subsidies to those in need to assure that they can obtain at least basic health care coverage. It could do this better than it is doing today.

At the same time the government should *withdraw from* those activities that it is *not well suited to perform* — the regulation of industry prices and restrictions of entry placed on providers and facilities. The private sector, not government, should make the basic decisions on resource allocation. To assure that competition works fairly, however, government must fashion a more complete and equitable safety net.

Appendix

Current Policies to Finance Indigent Care

Medical indigence leads to uncompensated health care, encompassing a mixture of different kinds of care provided to different kinds of people. One kind of care is the charity care provided to the uninsured poor; nationally, however, the poor make up only about a third of those who lack health insurance. Indeed, half of the uninsured are members of families with incomes that are at least twice the poverty level; and at least 75 percent of the uninsured are either employed (25 percent of them full time) or dependents of the employed, although some of them earn less than a poverty-level income.

Basically, medical indigency is the inability of a household to cover whatever medical bills it is responsible for on an out-of-pocket basis. Even routine medical expenses may be beyond the means of an uninsured family. The problem of medical indigence is not exclusively a matter of having no insurance or no job, although these factors surely contribute to the problem. Many people with insurance coverage are vulnerable to high medical expenses, and some people with basic insurance coverage generate bad debts by failing to meet their front-end cost obligations (i.e., deductibles and copayments). This applies to Medicare recipients as well. Others who have insurance exhaust their benefits and cannot cover the back-end expenses. This happens when state caps on covered hospital days and dollar limits on covered outpatient care are exceeded under Medicaid, or when Medicare patients become responsible for 25 percent of their hospital bills after sixty days of hospitalization. It also happens under private insurance because of insufficient protection against the cost of catastrophic illness.

An estimated 31 to 37 million Americans lack insurance coverage. According to one recent estimate, about 9 percent of the population lacked health insurance throughout the year in 1984. When those who are uninsured only part of the year were included, this figure jumped to about 27 percent.[1]

Uncompensated care is a mixture of a large number of relatively small bills for such procedures as labor and delivery and outpatient care and a smaller number of very expensive major medical procedures such as neonatal care or intensive care.

The Annual Survey of Hospitals conducted by the American Hospital Association showed that community hospitals provided $6.2 billion in uncompensated care in 1982, or about 6 percent of the approximately $100 billion in hospital payments.[2] Of this total, $4.5 billion resulted from bad debts and $1.7 billion from provision of charity care. More recent estimates placed the total amount of uncompensated care at $7.4 billion in 1985. The burden of providing unpaid care is not distributed evenly across types of hospitals. For example, public teaching hospitals bear a disproportionately large share; according to one study, they accounted for three times as much uncompensated care as their share of all hospital charges.[3]

A wide variety of federal and state programs is currently available to provide and finance health care for the medically indigent.

MEDICAID

Medicaid is a federal-state insurance program that pays for medical services for certain low-income groups. It is administered by the states under federal guidelines that establish eligibility criteria, the benefits covered, and the methods of paying providers. The federal government provides matching grants to the states that range from 50 to 78 percent of the total expenditures.

Certain basic health care services must be offered in any state Medicaid program, including inpatient hospital care, outpatient care, laboratory and X ray services, and skilled nursing facility and physician services. States may limit the scope of such services, for example, by restricting the number of days of hospital coverage Medicaid will pay for or the number of covered outpatient visits. Optional services include prescription drugs and dental care.

The combined federal-state spending for Medicaid totaled $47 billion in fiscal 1986. Nevertheless, only about half of the poor are eligible for Medicaid, down from about two-thirds a decade ago. There are two basic routes to Medicaid eligibility: through eligibility for the AFDC program and through the SSI program. AFDC is a cash-assistance program for poor families with children, and SSI is a cash-assistance program for the elderly poor, the disabled, and the blind. Thus, eligibility for government-provided health assistance for low-income households hinges on prior eligibility for basic government welfare programs. The inequities and imbalances in the welfare system are transported directly into subsidies for health care. This stands in sharp contrast with Medicare, where eligibility depends on age alone.

Recent federal legislation permits states to offer Medicaid coverage to households that are poor but ineligible for cash assistance under AFDC or

SSI. But few states have moved to extend coverage under this voluntary arrangement.

Although it is difficult to establish a precise link between eligibility for Medicaid coverage and health status, studies have uncovered correlations that *suggest* a positive relationship. Certainly, access to and use of the health care system by the poor began to improve after Medicaid and Medicare were enacted in 1965.

OTHER FEDERAL PROGRAMS

Some special features of federal programs serve a segment of the population that is categorically ineligible for Medicaid through AFDC or SSI participation. This group, which includes intact families, single adults, and childless couples, can receive federal aid under certain circumstances. For example, if a woman is pregnant with her first child or if a two-parent household with one worker has a child five years of age or younger, coverage may be available at the state's option. (In this case, the child is covered if the household otherwise meets the income and asset criteria for Medicaid eligibility.) Some states had this kind of coverage and some did not in 1984, when Congress (in the Deficit Reduction Act) mandated the Medicaid eligibility of these two categories of households that would otherwise be ineligible even though their incomes were low enough to qualify. The federal government essentially converted an optionally categorically needy approach into a mandatory categorically needy approach, in effect expanding coverage somewhat under the regular Medicaid program.

Another optionally categorically needy group is households headed by an unemployed parent. About half of the states have covered such families under AFDC and thereby made them eligible for Medicaid.

Thus, one direction Medicaid expansion can take at the state level is *across* types of households that fall below income and asset cutoff lines. This would pick up some of the people who are poor but were previously knocked out of the federal-state safety net because of their family or work status.

A second type of expansion would extend *upward* into the income distribution. This would be accomplished principally through the medically needy program. This type of program, which is optional for the states, also involves matching federal money. Thirty states now have medically needy programs. People qualify for assistance if their incomes are up to 133 percent of the state's AFDC payment standard but their medical expenses in a given year cause them to "spend down" into the regular Medicaid category. The payment standard establishes eligibility for AFDC and the maximum

AFDC benefits that the state will pay if a household has no other income. Although the actual income of medically needy people is somewhat above the AFDC payment standard, their adjusted income, net of medical expenses, would be under this standard.

In the 1981 Omnibus Budget Reconciliation Act, Congress authorized the states to establish limited medically needy programs that offer some of the mandatory health services covered by Medicaid. States can extend pre-natal and delivery services to poor pregnant women and ambulatory care to children without providing complete medically indigent coverage to such groups as the elderly and the disabled.

Aside from Medicaid, which provides insurance coverage, the federal government offers a series of block grants to states that directly finance health care services, including maternal and child health, preventive care, primary care, and Indian Health Centers. Together, these grants account for about $1.5 billion a year in federal outlays.

The Maternal and Child Health Services program is a state-adminis-tered effort that provides prenatal, delivery, and postpartum care to low-income women who are ineligible for Medicaid. The primary-care program supports community health centers in areas designated as underserved.

The federal government has also supported the provision of charity care through the Hill-Burton program. Hospitals that received Hill-Burton funds supporting the construction or modernization of facilities took on a twenty-year obligation to provide some charity care, and many hospitals are still fulfilling this obligation.

STATE-ONLY PROGRAMS

Some people ineligible for Medicaid are covered exclusively with state funding through several types of state-only programs. (See "The South Caro-lina Approach," page 106.) One type enables high-risk individuals whose actuarially determined health insurance premiums would be unaffordable to buy into a risk-sharing program that brings the costs down to a practical level. Pooling arrangements of this kind are now incorporated in programs in Connecticut, Florida, Indiana, Minnesota, and North Dakota.

Another type is a catastrophic expense program which picks up the costs of serious and expensive illnesses that exceed some out-of-pocket limit. Under these programs, with which Alaska, Rhode Island, and Maine have experimented, the state effectively offers stop-loss insurance protec-tion to people who have medical bills that far exceed their insurance cover-age and a measure of assistance to those who are uninsured.

States also provide funding for indigent care through their taxing

106

authority, which can generate revenues that are rechanneled to hospitals with particularly large shares of uncompensated care. Surcharges on hospital revenues are used to fund risk pools for such hospitals in New York and Florida. There are important differences between these two efforts. Florida taxes hospital net revenues, whereas New York taxes insurance premiums. Thus, the Florida approach captures some revenue from self-insured companies that would not be collected under the New York model. Also, the Florida model does not combine the indigent care tax with state hospital rate setting, whereas New York uses the two approaches in tandem.

In Nevada and Oklahoma, indigent care pools are funded through property taxes. Indigent care task forces in Ohio and Arkansas have also recommended the establishment of such pools. In Arkansas, the task force recommended funding through tax assessments on smoking and gambling.

THE SOUTH CAROLINA APPROACH

In 1985, the South Carolina General Assembly passed the South Carolina Medically Indigent Assistance Act. This legislation increased access to health care in three ways.

First, by combining state funds and matching federal dollars, the state has added an estimated 42,600 poor people to AFDC and Medicaid. This was accomplished by raising eligibility standards from an annual income of $2,748 to $5,325 for a family of four, or from 27 percent to 50 percent of the federal poverty guidelines. The state has required implementation of the AFDC Unemployed Parent program covering low-income two-parent families where a parent is unemployed.

Second, the bill created the Medically Indigent Assistance Fund, which increased access to care by creating a pool of funds to cover people whose incomes are above the AFDC-Medicaid eligibility standard but who cannot afford hospitalization. This fund became operational on January 1, 1986, and is financed equally by county governments and general hospitals.

Third, hospitals are prohibited from denying emergency admissions based on ability to pay or county of residence.

The bill combines these steps to improve access with a series of new initiatives designed to build more cost discipline into both the Medicaid program and the overall hospital market. It provides cost-containment incentives for providers of care by converting the Medicaid hospital reimbursement system to a prospective payment system. Other measures incorporated into the Medicaid program require utilization reviews for appropriateness of treatment and length of stay, preadmission certification of nonemergency admissions, mandatory outpatient surgery in appropriate cases, and a pilot study of second surgical opinions.

All-payer rate setting systems are also used to fund indigent care. These systems attempt to put all payers — government, commercial insurers, Blue Cross, and self-insured employers — on an equal footing through establishing indigent care pools that rechannel funds from hospitals with relatively low proportions of bad debts and charity to those with a disproportionately high share of uncompensated care. In Maryland, Massachusetts, New Jersey, and New York, state rate-setting commissions set higher allowable rates for hospitals with large amounts of bad debt and charity.

All fifty states have programs that reimburse health care providers for care given to specified groups ineligible for Medicaid. These programs include the variety array of state general-relief efforts and have diverse target populations. Some are funded only by states, some only by counties, and some on a joint state-county basis. Other programs are special needs efforts targeted to certain groups in need or to certain diseases or conditions such as hemophilia, speech and hearing problems, and vision problems. States usually fund these programs without county support.

This complex array of federal, state, and local initiatives has provided a considerable amount of help to the poor and has often averted or ameliorated the most egregious inequities. Nevertheless, any patchwork approach inevitably leads to inequities involving people who fall through the cracks. Clearly, this review of government programs shows that public subsidies for the health care of the poor are substantial. But there are still many holes in our health care safety net.

ENDNOTES

CHAPTER 1

1. See U.S. Chamber of Commerce, *Employee Benefits, 1984* (Washington, D.C.: U.S. Chamber of Commerce, 1986).

CHAPTER 2

1. *Economic Report of the President, 1985* (Washington, D.C.: U.S. Government Printing Office, 1985), p. 133; "National Health Expenditures, 1985," *Health Care Financing Review* 8: 1 (Fall 1986), p. 1.

2. U.S. Office of Management and Budget, *Budget of the U.S. Government, FY 1987* (Washington, D.C.: U.S. Government Printing Office, 1985), pp. 5-101.

3. Amy K. Taylor and Gail R. Wilensky, "The Effect of Tax Policies on Expenditures for Private Health Insurance," in *Market Reforms in Health Care: Current Issues, New Directions, Strategic Decisions*, ed. Jack A. Meyer (Washington, D.C.: American Enterprise Institute, 1983), p. 165.

4. See U.S. Chamber of Commerce, *Employee Benefits, 1984* (Washington, D.C.: U.S. Chamber of Commerce, 1986).

5. Mark S. Freeland and Carol Ellen Schendler, "Health Spending in the 1980s: Integration of Clinical Practice Patterns with Management," *Health Care Financing Review* (Spring 1984), Table 7, pp. 54-55.

6. National Center for Health Statistics, *Health: United States, 1983*, DHHS Pub. No. (PHS) 84-1232, Public Health Service (Washington, D.C.: U.S. Government Printing Office, December 1983), Tables 55 - 58, pp. 161-172.

7. National Center for Health Statistics, *Health: United States, 1983*, Table 61 and Table 62, pp. 169 and 171.

8. Making employee benefits a mandatory subject of collective bargaining was established under judicial interpretations of the National Labor Relations Act, while the Internal Revenue Code of 1954 permitted employees to exclude the full amount of their employer's contribution to health insurance from their taxable income.

9. See Pamela J. Farley and Daniel C. Walden, *Private Insurance and Public Programs: Coverage of Health Services* (Washington, D.C.: U.S. Department of Health and Human Services, photocopy, 1985), p. 16.

10. National Center for Health Statistics, *Health: United States, 1983*, p. 137.

11. Alan C. Monheit, Michael M. Hagan, Marc L. Berk, and Pamela J. Farley, "The Employed Uninsured and the Role of Public Policy" (paper presented at Annual Meeting of the American Public Health Association, photocopy, November 13, 1984).

12. Alan C. Monheit, Michael M. Hagan, Marc L. Berk, and Gail R. Wilensky, "Health Insurance for the Unemployed: Is Federal Legislation Needed?" in *Health Affairs* 3: 1 (Spring 1984).

13. Monheit, Hagan, Berk, and Farley, "The Employed Uninsured," pp. 31-32.

14. Susan Blank with Thomas Brock, "Health, Health Care, and Economic Self-Sufficiency," in *Charting the Future of Health Care: Policy, Politics, and Public Health,* eds. Jack A. Meyer and Marion Ein Lewin (Washington, D.C.: American Enterprise Institute, 1987), p. 165.

15. Robert J. Blendon and Thomas W. Maloney, *New Approaches to the Medicaid Crisis* (New York: F & S Press, 1982), p. 12.

16. *Aging in America: Trends and Projections* (Washington, D.C.: U.S. Senate Special Committee on Aging and the American Association of Retired Persons, 1984), pp. 22-24.

17. *Economic Report of the President, 1985*, p. 136.

18. U.S. Special Committee on Aging in conjunction with the American Association of Retired Persons, the Federal Council on the Aging, and the Administration on Aging, *Aging America: Trends and Projections*, 1985-86 Edition, Series P-25 (Washington, D.C.: U.S. Department of Health and Human Services, 1986), Chart 1-2, p. 11.

CHAPTER 3

1. "Bad Debt and Charity Care in Registered Community Hospitals, 1979-1982," *Hospitals* (October 16, 1984).

2. Committee on Implications of For-Profit Enterprise in Health Care, Division of Health Care Services, *For-Profit Enterprise in Health Care* (Washington, D.C.: Institute of Medicine, National Academy Press, 1986).

3. See Commentary of Joseph P. Newhouse in *A New Approach to the Economics of Health Care*, ed. Mancur Olson (Washington, D.C.: American Enterprise Institute, 1981), pp. 204-205.

4. Ingemar Stohl, "Can Equality and Efficiency be Combined? The Experience of the Planned Swedish Health Care System," in *A New Approach to the Economics of Health Care*, ed. Olson, pp. 172-195.

5. Bruce Steinwald and Frank A. Sloan, "Regulatory Approaches to Hospital Cost Containment: A Synthesis of Empirical Evidence," in *A New Approach to the Economics of Health Care*, ed. Olson, pp. 274-308.

CHAPTER 4

1. See Edward Berkowitz and Monroe Berkowitz, "Incentives for Reducing the Costs of Disability," an unpublished paper prepared for CED health care project, January 1986.

2. "Private Sector Health Care Innovations: Report on Survey of CED Trustee Organizations," an unpublished paper prepared for CED health care project, January 1986.

3. Amy K. Taylor and Gail R. Wilensky, "The Effect of Tax Policies on Expenditures for Private Health Insurance," in *Market Reforms in Health Care: Current Issues, New Directions, Strategic Decisions*, ed. Jack A. Meyer (Washington, D.C.: American Enterprise Institute, 1983), p. 165.

4. Interstudy, *National HMO Census, 1984*, p. 2.

5. The Equitable Life Assurance Society, *The Equitable Health Care Survey*, August 1983.

6. A. S. Hansen Company, *1983 Hansen Benefits Survey: Health Care Cost Containment Results*.

7. Judith Feder and William Scanlon, "Problems and Prospects in Financing Long-Term Care," an unpublished paper prepared for CED health care project, December 1986.

8. American Medical Association, *Socioeconomic Monitoring System Report*, November 1983.

9. Interstudy, *National HMO Census, 1984*, p. 3.

10. Interstudy, *National HMO Census, 1984*, p. 5.

11. Merton D. Finkler, "Changes in Certificate-of-Need Laws: Read the Fine Print," in *Incentives vs. Controls in Health Care: Broadening the Debate*, ed. Jack A. Meyer (Washington, D.C.: American Enterprise Institute, 1985), p. 136. See also Don E. Detmer, "Ambulatory Surgery," *New England Journal of Medicine* (December 1981), pp. 1406-9.

CHAPTER 5

1. The discussion of the implications of a regulated market for health care in this section is based on Ronald W. Hansen, "Stimulating Product Innovation and Reforming the Health Care Reimbursement System," an unpublished paper prepared for the CED health care project, 1986.

2. Mark S. Freeland and Carol E. Schendler, "Health Spending in the 1980s: Integration of Clinical Practice Patterns with Management," *Health Care Financing Review* 5: 3 (Spring 1984), pp. 39-41.

3. See William M. Wardell, Maureen S. May, and A. Gene Trimble, "New Drug Development by United States Pharmaceutical Firms," *Clinical Pharmacology and Therapeutics* 32: 4 (October 1982), pp. 407-417.

4. See Earl P. Steinberg and Robert M. Heyssel, "Research and Teaching in Medicine in a Market-Driven Health Care System," an unpublished paper prepared for the CED health care project, 1986, pp. 4-5.

5. See Paul J. Feldstein, *Health Care Economics* (New York: John Wiley & Sons, 1983), p. 400.

6. *Final Report on Technology Assessment and Coverage Decisionmaking in the Department of Health and Human Services* (Silver Springs, Maryland: Macro Systems, Inc., August 31, 1984). See also V. A. Bucci, J. B. Reiss, and N. C. Hall, "New Obstacles in the Path of Marketing New Medical Devices," *Health Care Technology* 2: 2 (Fall 1985).

7. Hansen, "Stimulating Product Innovation."

8. See William Wardell and Nancy Mattison, "The Potential for Pharmaceutical Development and Regulation," in *Meeting Human Needs*, ed. Jack A. Meyer (Washington, D.C.: American Enterprise Institute, 1982), pp. 383-404.

9. William M. Wardell, "The History of Drug Discovery, Development, and Regulation," in *Issues in Pharmaceutical Economics*, ed. R. I. Chien (Lexington, Massachusetts: Lexington Books, 1979), pp. 3-11.

10. Ronald W. Hansen, "The Pharmaceutical Development Process: Estimates of Development Costs and Times and the Effects of Proposed Regulatory Changes," in *Issues in Pharmaceutical Economics*, ed. R. I. Chien, pp. 151-187.

11. These estimates include the clinical and preclinical costs for both successful and unsuccessful compounds, as well as the time-cost of the R&D investment during the study and regulatory assessment periods and the effects of inflation.

12. *Economic Costs of FDA Regulations* (Washington, D.C.: Pharmaceutical Manufacturers Association, 1981); U. S. General Accounting Office, *FDA Drug Approval — A Lengthy Process that Delays the Availability of Important New Drugs*, HRD-80-64, May 28, 1980; William M. Wardell, "Introduction of New Therapeutic Drugs in the United States and Great Britain: An International Comparison," *Clinical Pharmacology and Therapeutics*: 14 (1983), pp. 773-790.

13. Henry Grabowski and John Vernon, "A Sensitivity Analysis of Expected Profitability of Pharmaceutical Research and Development," *Managerial and Decision Economics*, Vol. 3 (1982), pp. 36-40; Prafulla Joglekar and Morton L. Paterson, "A Closer Look at the Returns and Risks of Pharmaceutical R & D," *Journal of Health Economics*, Vol. 5 (1986), pp. 153-177; John R. Virts and J. Fred Weston, "Expectations and the Allocation of Research and Development Resources," in *Drugs and Health*, ed. R. Helms (Washington, D.C.: American Enterprise Institute, 1981), pp. 21-45.

CHAPTER 6

1. See, for example, Bruce Steinwald and Frank A. Sloan, "Regulatory Approaches to Hospital Cost Containment: A Synthesis of Empirical Evidence," in *A New Approach to the Economics of Health Care*, ed. M. Olson, pp. 274-308.

2. Frank A. Sloan, Janet Mitchell, and Jerry Cromwell, "Physician Participation in State Medicaid Programs," *Journal of Human Resources*, XIII Supplement (1978), pp. 211-241.

3. Alain C. Enthoven, *Health Plan* (Boston, Massachusetts: Addison-Wesley Press, 1980), pp. 114-144.

4. Congressional Budget Office, *Reducing Poverty Among Children* (Washington, D.C.: U.S. Government Printing Office, May 1985), pp. 34-56.

5. Congressional Budget Office, *Reducing Poverty Among Children*, p. 35.

6. Congressional Budget Office, *Reducing Poverty Among Children*, p. 57.

7. Congressional Budget Office, *Reducing the Deficit: Spending and Revenue Options*, A Report to the Senate and House Committees on the Budget, Part II (Washington, D.C.: U.S. Government Printing Office, January 1987), pp. 241-242.

8. Congressional Budget Office, *Reducing the Deficit*, p. 87.

9. The objective is to place no greater upward pressure on interest rates, which requires that there be no net increase in the government's borrowing requirement. A slightly larger surplus in the Old Age and Survivors Insurance or Hospital Insurance trust funds would be used to purchase Treasury bills and bonds. If the buildup in such funds is equivalent to the additional general revenues spent, the government would be internally financing the added spending and should not have to borrow additional funds from the private sector. Because our concern is to avoid putting any new pressure on the pool of private savings arising from greater government debt, our focus may transcend the boundaries of the trust funds without violating those boundaries in any way.

10. Congressional Budget Office, *Reducing the Deficit*, p. 94.

APPENDIX

1. Pamela J. Farley, "Who are the Uninsured?" in *Milbank Memorial Fund Quarterly/Health and Society* 63: 3 (1985), p. 477.

2. Frank A. Sloan, Joseph Valvona, and Ross Mullner, "Identifying the Issues: A Statistical Profile," in *Uncompensated Hospital Care: Rights and Responsibilities* (Baltimore, Maryland: Johns Hopkins University Press, 1986).

3. Sloan, Valvona, and Mullner, "Identifying the Issues."

Memoranda of Comment, Reservation, or Dissent

Page 22, FRANKLIN A. LINDSAY, with which Harold A. Poling and Elmer B. Staats have asked to be associated.

Health care is probably the only major service still measured primarily by inputs rather than outputs. But in spite of the obvious difficulties, a greater effort should be made by public and private health care administrators to develop measures of output, including both quantitative and qualitative (quality of life) measures. Measures of quality of outputs are prerequisites for improvement in the quality of health care and the control of the level of resources devoted to health care. Because, unlike manufacturing, so much of health care is in the form of services, the higher the utilization the higher the cost.

Following is a list of background research papers prepared in association with the work of the CED Subcommittee on Health Care Policy. The papers will be published in a separate volume.

Incentives for Reducing the Costs of Disability
Edward Berkowitz, Director, Program in History and Public Policy, The George Washington University; and Monroe Berkowitz, Chairman, Department of Economics, and Director, Bureau of Economic Research, Rutgers University

Access to Advanced Medical Techniques
Douglas Besharov, School of Law, College of William and Mary, and Visiting Scholar, American Enterprise Institute; and Jessica Silver, Visiting Fellow, American Enterprise Institute

Market Incentives and the Costs of Medical Malpractice
Patricia M. Danzon, Associate Professor, Health Care Systems and Insurance Departments, The Wharton School, University of Pennsylvania

Problems and Prospects in Financing Long-Term Care
Judith Feder, Co-Director, Center for Health Policy Studies, Georgetown University; and William J. Scanlon, Co-Director, Center for Health Policy Studies, Georgetown University

Stimulating Product Innovation and Reforming the Health Care Reimbursement System
Ronald W. Hansen, Associate Merrell Dow Professorship, Division of Pharmaceutical Administration, Ohio State University
(The paper was prepared while Mr. Hansen was Associate Director of the Center for Research and Government Policy and Business at the University of Rochester.)

What Employers Can Do About Medical Care Costs: Managing Health and Productivity
Jeffrey S. Harris, Director of Health and Safety, Northern Telecom Inc.

Medical Research and Teaching in A Market-Driven Health Care System
Robert M. Heyssel, President, Johns Hopkins Hospital; and Earl P. Steinberg, Professor, The Johns Hopkins School of Medicine, Johns Hopkins Hospital

Improving the Role of Private Markets in Financing Long-Term Care Services
Mark R. Meiners, Senior Research Manager, Long-Term Care, National Center for Health Services Research; and Jay Neil Greenberg, Director, Long-Term Care Group, Health Policy Center, Heller Graduate School, Brandeis University

OBJECTIVES OF THE COMMITTEE FOR ECONOMIC DEVELOPMENT

For over forty years, the Committee for Economic Development has been a respected influence on the formation of business and public policy. CED is devoted to these two objectives:

To develop, through objective research and informed discussion, findings and recommendations for private and public policy that will contribute to preserving and strengthening our free society, achieving steady economic growth at high employment and reasonably stable prices, increasing productivity and living standards, providing greater and more equal opportunity for every citizen, and improving the quality of life for all.

To bring about increasing understanding by present and future leaders in business, government, and education, and among concerned citizens, of the importance of these objectives and the ways in which they can be achieved.

CED's work is supported strictly by private voluntary contributions from business and industry, foundations, and individuals. It is independent, nonprofit, nonpartisan, and nonpolitical.

The two hundred trustees, who generally are presidents or board chairmen of corporations and presidents of universities, are chosen for their individual capacities rather than as representatives of any particular interests. By working with scholars, they unite business judgment and experience with scholarship in analyzing the issues and developing recommendations to resolve the economic problems that constantly arise in a dynamic and demographic society.

Through this business-academic partnership, CED endeavors to develop policy statements and other research materials that command themselves as guides to public and business policy; that can be used as texts in college economics and political science courses and in management training courses; that will be considered and discussed by newspaper and magazine editors, columnists, and commentators; and that are distributed abroad to promote better understanding of the American economic system.

CED believes that by enabling businessmen to demonstrate constructively their concern for the general welfare, it is helping business to earn and maintain the national and community respect essential to the successful functioning of the free enterprise capitalist system.

STATEMENTS ON NATIONAL POLICY
ISSUED BY THE RESEARCH AND POLICY COMMITTEE

SELECTED PUBLICATIONS

Work and Change: Labor Market Adjustment Policies in a
  Competitive World *(1987)*

Leadership for Dynamic State Economies *(1986)*

Fighting Federal Deficits: The Time for Hard Choices *(1985)*

Strategy for U.S. Industrial Competitiveness *(1984)*

Strengthening the Federal Budget Process:
  A Requirement for Effective Fiscal Control *(1983)*

Productivity Policy: Key to the Nation's Economic Future *(1983)*

Energy Prices and Public Policy *(1982)*

Public-Private Partnership: An Opportunity for Urban Communities *(1982)*

Reforming Retirement Policies *(1981)*

Transnational Corporations and Developing Countries: New Policies for a
  Changing World Economy *(1981)*

Fighting Inflation and Rebuilding a Sound Economy *(1980)*

Stimulating Technological Progress *(1980)*

Helping Insure Our Energy Future:
  A Program for Developing Synthetic Fuel Plants Now *(1979)*

Redefining Government's Role in the Market System *(1979)*

Improving Management of the Public Work Force:
  The Challenge to State and Local Government *(1978)*

Jobs for the Hard-to-Employ:
  New Directions for a Public-Private Partnership *(1978)*

An Approach to Federal Urban Policy *(1977)*

Key Elements of a National Energy Strategy *(1977)*

The Economy in 1977–78: Strategy for an Enduring Expansion *(1976)*

Nuclear Energy and National Security *(1976)*

Fighting Inflation and Promoting Growth *(1976)*

Improving Productivity in State and Local Government *(1976)*

*International Economic Consequences of High-Priced Energy *(1975)*

Broadcasting and Cable Television:
  Policies for Diversity and Change *(1975)*

Achieving Energy Independence *(1974)*

A New U.S. Farm Policy for Changing World Food Needs *(1974)*

Congressional Decision Making for National Security *(1974)*

*Toward a New International Economic System:
  A Joint Japanese-American View *(1974)*

More Effective Programs for a Cleaner Environment *(1974)*

The Management and Financing of Colleges *(1973)*

Strengthening the World Monetary System *(1973)*

Financing the Nation's Housing Needs *(1973)*

Building a National Health-Care System *(1973)*

*A New Trade Policy Toward Communist Countries *(1972)*

High Employment Without Inflation:
  A Positive Program for Economic Stabilization *(1972)*

Reducing Crime and Assuring Justice *(1972)*

Military Manpower and National Security *(1972)*

The United States and the European Community:
  Policies for a Changing World Economy *(1971)*

Improving Federal Program Performance *(1971)*

Social Responsibilities of Business Corporations *(1971)*

Education for the Urban Disadvantaged:
  From Preschool to Employment *(1971)*

Further Weapons Against Inflation *(1970)*

Making Congress More Effective *(1970)*

Training and Jobs for the Urban Poor *(1970)*

Improving the Public Welfare System *(1970)*

Reshaping Government in Metropolitan Areas *(1970)*

Economic Growth in the United States *(1969)*

Assisting Development in Low-Income Countries *(1969)*

*Nontariff Distortions of Trade *(1969)*

Fiscal and Monetary Policies for Steady Economic Growth *(1969)*

Financing a Better Election System *(1968)*

Innovation in Education: New Directions for the American School *(1968)*

Modernizing State Government *(1967)*

*Trade Policy Toward Low-Income Countries *(1967)*

How Low Income Countries Can Advance Their Own Growth *(1966)*

*Statements issued in association with CED counterpart organizations in foreign countries.

CED COUNTERPART ORGANIZATIONS IN FOREIGN COUNTRIES

Close relations exist between the Committee for Economic Development and independent, nonpolitical research organizations in other countries. Such counterpart groups are composed of business executives and scholars and have objectives similar to those of CED, which they pursue by similarly objective methods. CED cooperates with these organizations on research and study projects of common interest to the various countries concerned. This program has resulted in a number of joint policy statements involving such international matters as energy, East-West trade, assistance to the developing countries, and the reduction of nontariff barriers to trade.

| CE | Círculo de Empresarios
Serrano Jover 5-2° Madrid 8, Spain |
| --- | --- |
| **CEDA** | Committee for Economic Development of Australia
139 Macquarie Street, Sydney 2001,
New South Wales, Australia |
| **CEPES** | Europäische Vereinigung für
Wirtschaftliche und Soziale Entwicklung
Reuterweg 14,6000 Frankfurt/Main, West Germany |
| **IDEP** | Institut de l'Entreprise
6, rue Clément-Marot, 75008 Paris, France |
| 経済同友会 | Keizai Doyukai
(Japan Committee for Economic Development)
Japan Industrial Club Bldg.
1 Marunouchi, Chiyoda-ku, Tokyo, Japan |
| **PSI** | Policy Studies Institute
100, Park Village East, London NW1 3SR, England |
| **SNS** | Studieförbundet Näringsliv och Samhälle
Sköldungagatan 2, 11427 Stockholm, Sweden |